Self-Assessment Color Review
Veterinary Cytology: Dog, Cat, Horse, and Cow
Second Edition

Self-Assessment Color Review

Veterinary Cytology: Dog, Cat, Horse, and Cow

Second Edition

Francesco Cian
DVM, DipECVCP, FRCPath, MRCVS
RCVS Specialist in Veterinary Pathology (Clinical Pathology)
BattLab, University of Warwick Science Park
Coventry, Warwickshire, UK

Kathleen P. Freeman
DVM, BS, MS, PhD, DipECVCP, FRCPath, MRCVS
RCVS Specialist in Veterinary Pathology (Clinical Pathology)
IDEXX Laboratories, Ltd
Wetherby, West Yorkshire, UK

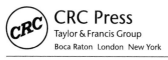

CRC Press
Taylor & Francis Group
Boca Raton London New York

CRC Press is an imprint of the
Taylor & Francis Group, an **informa** business

CRC Press
Taylor & Francis Group
6000 Broken Sound Parkway NW, Suite 300
Boca Raton, FL 33487-2742

© 2017 by Taylor & Francis Group, LLC
CRC Press is an imprint of Taylor & Francis Group, an Informa business

No claim to original U.S. Government works

Printed in the UK by Severn, Gloucester on responsibly sourced paper

 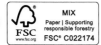

Version Date: 20160913

International Standard Book Number-13: 978-1-4987-6671-5 (Paperback)

Visit the Taylor & Francis Web site at
http://www.taylorandfrancis.com

and the CRC Press Web site at
http://www.crcpress.com

Contents

Preface to the first edition

This book aims to provide a representative sample of cytology cases encountered in a variety of diagnostic situations. It is not an inclusive text covering all conditions but offers a variety of cytology features and patterns from which anyone interested in veterinary cytology can continue to learn and test their knowledge. Bone marrow is covered by only a very few cases, since readers should not be misled and believe that they might be able to interpret a bone marrow from a single cytological field – they also need extensive knowledge and experience in haematology.

The format throughout the text encourages description and interpretation of the cytological specimens represented in the photomicrographs. The exercise of description is one that should not be ignored and, laborious as it may seem to those making their first attempts, it is critical for the development of a discriminating cytologist. The process of description provides a guide to a systematic method for covering the cellular and noncellular material that is present.

It is important to admit when cells or features are recognized but cannot be categorized. Knowledge of the range of 'normal' for various sites and types of specimens is critical. The recognition of normality provides the basis for recognition of deviations from 'normal' and the presence of disease. It is vitally important that the student of cytology strives to obtain and examine a variety of specimens that represent 'normal' for the age, system, physiological status, species, method of collection, method of cytological presentation and staining. Only by an appreciation of the range of presentations that can represent a 'normal' collection can one become comfortable with the various types of specimens and their interpretation.

The process of description itself is often helpful in arriving at a suitable interpretation. By taking time to describe, the mental process of discriminating between various broad categories of pathology and the more specific conditions that may occur at a particular site or with a particular species becomes a systematic process of inclusion or elimination.

Once the student of cytology becomes comfortable with the descriptive process, the ability to provide an interpretation, taking into account the description of the smear and the clinical history, also requires practice. One of the most common mistakes is to let the clinical history dictate the interpretation of the cytological specimen. The clinical history should provide a background from which interpretation should take some clues. One or several conditions or processes may be possible given a particular history, but there must also be strong cytological evidence for a particular interpretation before it can be given.

The degree of confidence that one has in the interpretation is also important. This may vary with experience and with the degree of clarity and correlation between the cytological specimen and the clinical history. The degree of certainty of the reporting cytologist is of crucial importance to the clinician, who can then balance the clinical appearance and history against the cytological description and interpretation to help determine a clinical or working diagnosis.

So, to those readers who wish to embark upon the journey of cytological exploration, I urge you to continue to strive to be true to the classic exercises of description and interpretation. Seek histological and/or clinical follow-up where and when it is appropriate. Continue to learn the fascinating science and art of cytological diagnosis.

Kathleen P. Freeman

Preface to the second edition

It has been ten years since the first edition of this book was published. Since then there has been an exponential increase in the interest for cytology, resulting in the publication of several textbooks on the topic. Our book is different from the others in several ways since it has been written with the idea of teaching cytology through clinical cases, with a practical and clinical approach. We believe this will be useful for all those general practitioners who deal with cytology on a daily basis, as well as for trainees in clinical pathology or anatomical pathology who are learning cytological interpretation.

In the words of the famous human cytopathologist, Richard Mac DeMay, "welcome to the world of the art and science of cytopathology".

Francesco Cian
Kathleen P. Freeman

Acknowledgments

Being editor of this book represents something very important for me since it was the first cytology textbook I bought when I was still a student of veterinary medicine, and Kathleen Freeman was the first clinical pathologist I visited during my externship. She helped me to discover the beauty of veterinary clinical pathology, in the same way we hope to do with the readers of this book.

A special thanks goes to my family, who have always supported me in my life choices, and to the thousands of people from all over the world who have joined and supported the Veterinary Cytology Facebook page I created five years ago. We have exchanged a lot of cases and interesting information about cytology. I hope you will find this book an additional and valid support to your learning.

Francesco Cian

When the publishers approached me to do a second edition of this book with updated cases, I decided to find a keen young clinical pathologist to take over the main editing duties. Francesco Cian fitted the bill perfectly. I have worked with Francesco, first as a student and then as a colleague, over the past ten years and know him to be a very skilled and knowledgeable cytopathologist and am thrilled that he was willing to carry on encouraging and educating others to appreciate cytology in many ways, including this case book. I hope you will enjoy the second edition as much Francesco and I have in preparing it.

Kathleen P. Freeman

Picture acknowledgments

64b and 95b, courtesy of Heather Holloway
100a, courtesy of Elizabeth Welsh
1a, b, courtesy of Francesco Albanese
158c, courtesy of Roberta Rasotto

Contributors

First edition

A. Rick Alleman DVM, PhD,
  DipACVP, DipABVP
College of Veterinary Medicine
University of Florida
Gainesville, Florida, USA

Joan Duncan BVMS, PhD, FRCPath,
  CertVR, MRCVS
NationWide Laboratories
Poulton-le-Fylde, Lancashire, UK

Corinne Fournel-Fleury DVM, PhD,
  DipECVCP, HDR
Ecole Nationale Veterinaire de Lyon
Marcy L'Etoile, France

Kathleen P. Freeman DVM, BS,
  MS, PhD, DipECVCP, FRCPath,
  MRCVS
IDEXX Laboratories, Ltd.
Wetherby, West Yorkshire, UK

Karen L. Gerber BVSc(Pretoria),
  BVSc(Hons), DipACVP, MRCVS
Axiom Veterinary Laboratories
Newton Abbot, Devon, UK

J. Michael Harter DVM
Animal Medical Clinic
Rockford, Illinois, USA

Heather Holloway MA, VetMB,
  CertVC, DipRCPath, MRCVS
IDEXX Laboratories, Ltd.
Wetherby, West Yorkshire, UK

Hugh Larkin MVB, PhD, MRCPath,
  MECVCP, MRCVS
School of Veterinary Medicine
St George's University
Grenada, West Indies

Sally Lester DVM MVSc DipACVP
Central Laboratory for Veterinarians
Langley, British Columbia, Canada

Kostas Papasouliotis DVM, PhD,
  FRCPath, DipECVCP, MRCVS
School of Veterinary Science
University of Bristol
Langford, UK

Anne Lanevschi-Pietersma DVM, MS,
  DipACVP, ECVCP
Apartado 23
A Estrada 36680, Spain

Mark D. G. Pinches BVSc, MSc,
  MRCVS
School of Veterinary Science
University of Bristol
Langford, UK

Shashi K. Ramaiah DVM, PhD,
  DipACVP, DABT
Pfizer–Biotherapeutics Research
  Division
Cambridge, Massachusetts, USA

Federico Sacchini MVB, DipSCPCA,
  MPhil, DipECVCP, MRCVS
IDEXX Laboratories, Ltd.
Wetherby, West Yorkshire, UK

Elizabeth Villiers BVSc, DECVCP,
  FRCPath, CertSAM, CertVR,
  MRCVS
DWR Diagnostics
Six Mile Bottom, UK

Second edition (*additional contributors*)

Walter Bertazzolo DVM, DipECVCP
La Vallonèa Veterinary Diagnostic
    Laboratory, Alessano (LE), Italy
Clinical Laboratory, Animal Hospital
    "Città di Pavia"
Pavia, Italy

Ugo Bonfanti DVM, DipECVCP
La Vallonèa Veterinary Diagnostic
    Laboratory
Alessano (LE), Italy

**Francesco Cian DVM, FRCPath,
    DipECVCP, MRCVS**
RCVS Specialist in Veterinary
    Pathology (Clinical Pathology
BattLab
University of Warwick Science Park
Coventry, Warwickshire, UK

**Stefano Comazzi DVM, PhD,
    DipECVCP**
Department of Veterinary Medicine
University of Milan
Milan, Italy

Sharon M. Dial DVM, PhD, DACVP
Arizona Veterinary Diagnostic
    Laboratory
University of Arizona
Tucson, Arizona, USA

**Kathleen P. Freeman DVM, BS, MS,
    PhD, DipECVCP, MRCVS**
RCVS Specialist in Veterinary
    Pathology (Clinical Pathology)
IDEXX Laboratories, Ltd.
Wetherby, West Yorkshire, UK

**Emma Hooijberg BVSc, GPCert(SAP),
    DipECVCP**
Faculty of Veterinary Science
University of Pretoria
Pretoria, South Africa

Ernst Leidinger DVM, DipECVCP
Invitro Laboratories
Vienna, Austria

**Judith Leidinger DVM, FTA klin.
    Labordiagn**
Invitro Laboratories
Vienna, Austria

**Carlo Masserdotti DVM, DipECVCP,
    Spec Bioch Clin IAT**
IDEXX Laboratories, Ltd.
Milan, Italy

**Antonio Meléndez-Lazo DVM, MSc,
    DipECVCP, MRCVS**
LABOKLIN GmbH & Co.KG
Bad Kissingen, Germany

**Paola Monti DVM, MSc, FRCPath,
    DipACVP (Clinical Pathology)**
RCVS Specialist in Veterinary
    Pathology (Clinical Pathology)
DWR Diagnostics
Six Mile Bottom, UK

**Roger Powell MA, VetMB,
    DipRCPath, DipACVP (Clin. Path),
    FRCPath, MRCVS**
RCVS Specialist in Veterinary
    Pathology (Clinical Pathology)
PTDS Diagnostic Services
Hitchin, UK

Leslie C. Sharkey DVM, PhD, DipACVP
University of Minnesota
St Paul, Minnesota, USA

**Cathy Trumel DVM, PhD, DipECVCP,
    LCBM, CREFRE**
Université de Toulouse, INSERM,
    UPS, ENVT
Toulouse, France

**Tim Williams MA, VetMB, PhD,
    FRCPath, DipECVCP, MRCVS**
Department of Veterinary Medicine
University of Cambridge
Cambridge, UK

Abbreviations

ACTH	adrenocorticotrophic hormone	HDDS	high-dose dexamethasone suppression (test)
ALP	alkaline phosphatase	H&E	hematoxylin and eosin (stain)
ALT	alanine aminotransferase		
APTT	activated partial prothrombin time	LDDS	low-dose dexamethasone suppression (test)
AST	aspartate aminotransferase	MRI	magnetic resonance imaging
BIN	bronchial intraepithelial neoplasia	NADPH	nicotinamide adenine dinucleotide phosphate
BUN	blood urea nitrogen	N:C	nuclear:cytoplasmic (ratio)
CBC	complete blood count	NCC	nucleated cell count
CNS	central nervous system	NSAID	nonsteroidal anti-inflammatory drug
CSF	cerebrospinal fluid		
CT	computed tomography	PARR	PCR for antigen receptor rearrangement
DLH	domestic longhaired (cat)		
DSH	domestic shorthaired (cat)	PAS	periodic acid–Schiff (stain)
EDTA	ethylenediamine tetra-acetic acid	PCR	polymerase chain reaction
		PCV	packed cell volume
EGC	eosinophilic granuloma complex	PT	prothrombin time
		RBC	red blood cell
ELISA	enzyme-linked immunoabsorbent assay	RI	reference interval
		SCC	squamous cell carcinoma
FeLV	feline leukemia virus	SG	specific gravity
FIP	feline infectious peritonitis	TP	total protein
FIV	feline immunodeficiency virus	USG	urine specific gravity
FNA	fine needle aspirate	UV	ultraviolet
GGT	gamma glutamyl transferase	WBC	white blood cell

Conversion factors

	SI units	Conversion factor	Old units
Hematology			
PCV	l/l	0.01	%
RBCs	$\times 10^{12}$/l	1	$\times 10^6$/µl
Nucleated cell count	$\times 10^9$/l	1	$\times 10^3$/µl
Neutrophils	$\times 10^9$/l	1	$\times 10^3$/µl
Platelets	$\times 10^9$/l	1	$\times 10^3$/µl
Biochemistry/endocrinology			
ACTH	pmol/l	0.2222	pg/ml
Albumin	g/l	10	g/dl
Bilirubin	µmol/l	17.1	mg/dl
Cholesterol	mmol/l	0.0259	mg/dl
Cortisol	nmol/l	27.59	µg/dl
Creatinine	µmol/l	88.4	mg/dl
Globulin	g/l	10	g/dl
Glucose	mmol/l	0.0555	mg/dl
Total protein	g/l	10	g/dl
Total thyroxine (T4)	nmol/l	12.87	µg/dl
Triglyceride	mmol/l	0.0113	mg/dl
Urea nitrogen	mmol/l	0.357	mg/dl

Broad classification of cases

Body cavity fluids
5, 10, 11, 18, 55, 70, 71, 82, 100, 103,
127, 131, 135, 147, 149, 163

Ear and nose
12, 17, 31, 56, 59, 153

Endocrine system
19, 23, 35, 46, 138

Gastrointestinal system
4, 8, 47, 75, 81, 101

General interpretation
16, 22, 57, 58, 107, 118, 130, 134,
158

Hematopoietic system
25, 44, 49, 53, 62, 74, 76, 79, 84,
92, 94, 96, 98, 114, 119, 124, 155,
157, 159

Liver
26, 29, 48, 60, 64, 65, 67, 69, 80, 88,
106, 148, 151, 161

Mammary glands
39, 91, 164

Musculoskeletal system
2, 28, 66, 68, 78, 89, 129

Nervous system
6, 20, 102, 122, 143, 156

Reproductive system
15, 51, 87, 113, 139, 140, 162

Respiratory system
21, 27, 38, 43, 45, 52, 63, 86, 90, 112,
115, 116, 117, 137

Skin
1, 3, 7, 9, 13, 14, 30, 32, 33, 34, 36, 37,
40, 41, 42, 54, 72, 73, 83, 85, 93, 97,
99, 105, 108, 109, 111, 120, 121, 123,
125, 126, 132, 133, 136, 141, 144, 145,
150, 152, 154, 160, 165, 166

Urogenital system
24, 50, 77, 95, 104, 110, 128, 142, 146

CASE 1 An 18-month-old male Siamese cat was referred for multiple cutaneous and subcutaneous nodules that had only recently appeared. These were located on the trunk and left lip and on the fore- and hindlimbs. They measured approximately 2 cm in diameter and appeared rounded, smooth, and alopecic. Note the round, alopecic area on the left upper lip (**1a**). Multiple FNAs were obtained. A smear of one of the aspirates is shown (**1b**; May–Grünwald–Giemsa, ×40).

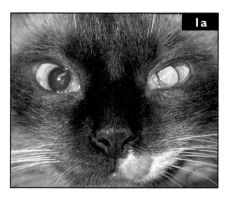
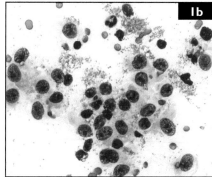

1 Identify the cell population present in the smear.
2 What is your interpretation?

CASE 2 A mass on the paw of a 9-year-old neutered male Labrador Retriever is aspirated. Smears of the aspirate are shown (**2a, b**; both Wright–Giemsa, ×50 oil).

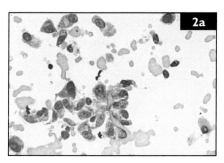
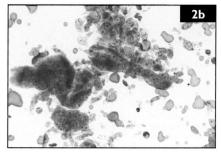

1 Describe the cells seen.
2 What is your cytologic interpretation?
3 What differential diagnoses would you consider?

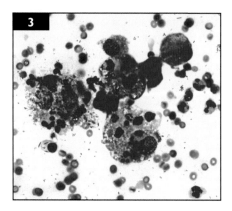

CASE 3 A 5-year-old neutered male Dachshund was referred for investigation of a raised skin lesion on the neck area. An FNA sample was collected and submitted for analysis. A smear of the sample is shown (3; Wright Giemsa, ×100 oil).

1 What process is observed in the photomicrograph?

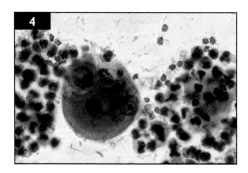

CASE 4 A 12-year-old Thoroughbred-cross gelding presented with a history of chronic weight loss. He had a poor coat and was emaciated at the time of referral. A peritoneal fluid specimen was submitted for body fluid analysis (erythrocyte count = 20×10^9/l; NCC = 15×10^9/l; TP = 32 g/l) and cytologic evaluation (4; Papanicolaou, ×100 oil). The RIs for equine (and bovine) pleural and abdominal fluid are shown below.

Category	TP	NCC
Transudate	<15 g/l	<5 × 10⁹/l
Modified transudate	5–35 g/l	<15 × 10⁹/l
Exudate	>35 g/l	>10 × 10⁹/l

1 How would you classify this fluid?
2 What cell types can be seen in the photomicrograph?
3 What is your interpretation?

CASE 5 This straw colored ascitic fluid (5a) was obtained by abdominocentesis from a 2-year-old cat with a history of pyrexia and abdominal distension. Photomicrographs of the fluid are shown (5b, c; Wright–Giemsa, ×50 oil and ×100 oil, respectively). Laboratory data for the fluid revealed: TP = 65.5 g/l; SG = 1.042; NCC = 0.43×10^9/l; RBCs = 0.01×10^{12}/l. Given the high fluid protein concentration, electrophoresis was requested (5d).

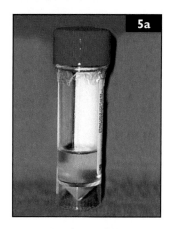
5a

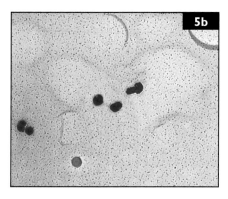
5b

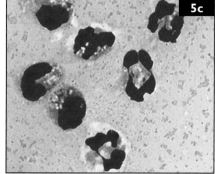
5c

1 Classify the fluid based on the photomicrographs and the laboratory data.
2 Interpret the electrophoresis trace.
3 Although the electrophoresis pattern is not pathognomonic for specific conditions, in the context of the other findings in this particular case, what diagnosis should be at the top of the differential list?

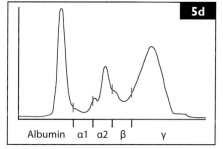
5d
Albumin   α1   α2   β   γ

3

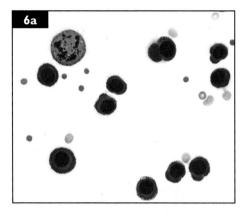

CASE 6 An 8 year-old spayed female Springer Spaniel was presented as an emergency for investigation of progressive ataxia of all four limbs, staggering, and behavioral changes. The dog had a solid mammary carcinoma surgically removed one year before. Neurologic examination and MRI indicated multifocal brain localization. A CSF sample was collected aseptically from the cisterna magna and revealed: total NCC = 30 cells/µl (RI = 0–6 cells/µl); RBCs = 90 cells/µl; protein = 0.25 g/l (RI = <0.35 g/l). A smear of the sample is shown (6a; Wright–Giemsa, ×50 oil).

1 Describe the cells shown in the photomicrograph.
2 What are your differential diagnoses based on these cytologic findings, and what additional tests would you recommend?

CASE 7 A firm ulcerated mass is noted on the jaw of a Friesian cow (7a). An FNA is collected. A smear of the aspirate is shown (7b; Wright–Giemsa, ×100 oil).

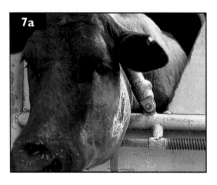
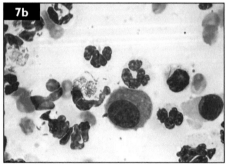

1 What cells are present?
2 What is your interpretation?

CASE 8 A 16-week-old female Husky-cross presented for persistent diarrhea. A fecal smear is shown (8; Gram, ×100 oil).

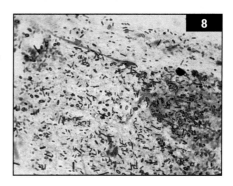

1 Describe the organisms seen.
2 Are the spore-forming gram-positive rods likely to be *Clostridium perfringens*?

CASE 9 A 6-year-old entire male Dalmatian was referred for evaluation of a slowly growing small cutaneous nodule on the left carpal region. A smear from the nodule is shown (9; Wright–Giemsa, ×50 oil).

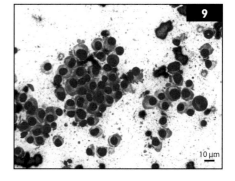

1 Describe the findings seen in the photomicrograph.
2 What is your interpretation?

CASE 10 Abdominal fluid is aspirated from a 5-year-old entire male Beagle. A smear of the sediment from the fluid is shown (10; Wright–Giemsa, ×50 oil).

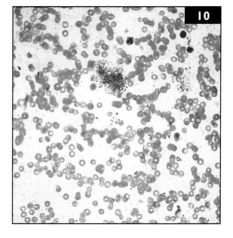

1 What features are shown?
2 What is the significance of these findings in an abdominal effusion?

CASE 11 A 19-year-old neutered male DSH cat presented with a history of lethargy and anorexia. On clinical examination, a cranial intra-abdominal mass was palpated; ultrasound examination revealed a small amount of free fluid and confirmed the presence of a 3 cm × 3 cm cranial intra-abdominal mass. A concentrated smear from the free fluid was made and submitted for cytologic analysis (**11a, b**; Wright–Giemsa, ×20 and ×50 oil, respectively).

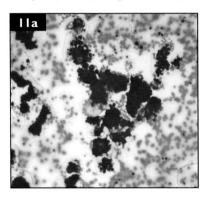
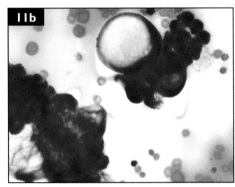

1 What is the most likely origin of the cell population?
2 Which criteria of malignancy do these cells demonstrate?
3 What is your interpretation of these findings?

CASE 12 A cat presents with ulceration and bleeding from the ear and side of the face (**12a**). An FNA is collected. A smear of the aspirate is shown (**12b**; Wright–Giemsa, ×100 oil).

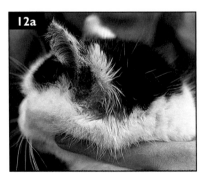
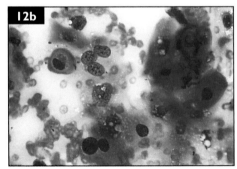

1 What cells are present?
2 What are your differential diagnoses?

CASE 13 A 12-year-old British Warmblood mare was presented for evaluation of a small cutaneous lesion at the level of the saddle. The mass was soft, nonalopecic, nodular, well-circumscribed, and approximately 2–3 cm in diameter. Fine needle aspiration of the mass was performed. Smears of the aspirate are shown (13a, b; Wright–Giemsa, ×50 oil and ×100 oil, respectively).

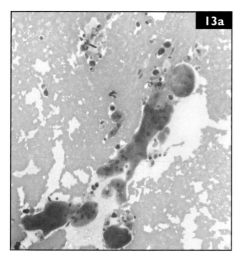
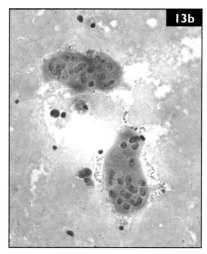

1 Describe the cells shown in the photomicrographs.
2 What are your differential diagnoses based on these cytologic findings?

CASE 14 A 6-year-old Golden Retriever has a rapidly growing, ill-defined mass above the left hock. The mass is subcutaneous and appears to extend circumferentially around the limb. The overlying skin is erythematous and beginning to ulcerate. An FNA is obtained and a smear made (14; Giemsa, ×100 oil).

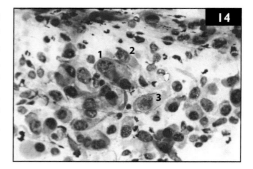

1 Describe and classify the cells illustrated.
2 What criteria of malignancy are present?
3 Can you suggest a likely diagnosis?

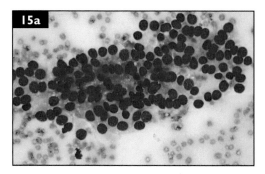

15a

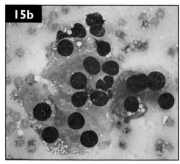

15b

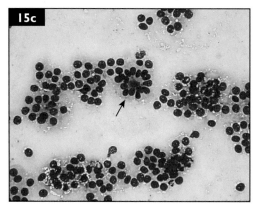

15c

CASE 15 A 10-year-old entire female Boxer presented with a history of persistent estrus and a hemorrhagic vulvar discharge. Abdominal ultrasound revealed a 7 cm left ovarian solid mass. An FNA from the ovarian mass was collected. Smears of the aspirate are shown (**15a–c**; Diff-Quik®, ×20, ×40, and ×10, respectively).

1 Identify the cell population present in the smear, and describe the most relevant characteristics.
2 What differential diagnoses would you consider for an ovarian mass?
3 What is your final interpretation?

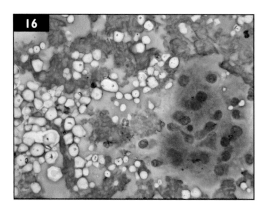

16

CASE 16 Identify the exogenous and possible foreign body material in this photomicrograph (**16**; Wright–Giemsa, ×50 oil).

CASE 17 A 13-year-old cat was presented with a smooth nodular lesion in the external ear canal. Direct smears of the contents were made (**17a, b**; Wright–Giemsa, ×40 and ×100 oil, respectively).

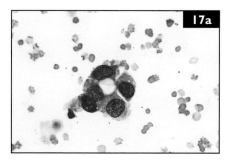 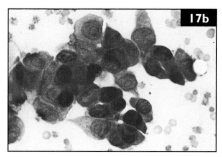

1 Describe the cells present.
2 What is the cell line of origin of these cells?
3 Are there features present that suggest malignancy?

CASE 18 A 12-year-old female DSH cat was presented for 2 weeks of anorexia and occasional episodes of vomiting. Abdominal ultrasound showed a well-defined, 4 cm mesenteric mass and a moderate abdominal effusion. Ultrasound-guided FNAs from the abdominal mass were obtained under sedation. Smears of the aspirates are shown (**18a, b**; Wright–Giemsa, ×20 and ×100 oil, respectively).

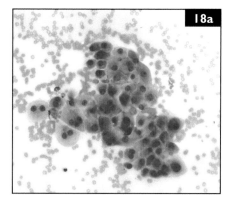

1 Describe the cells shown in the photomicrographs.
2 What are your differential diagnoses based on these cytologic findings, and what additional tests would you recommend?

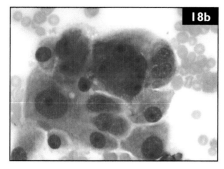

CASE 19 A 12-year-old neutered male DSH cat presented with polyuria and polydipsia, polyphagia, a pendulous abdomen, muscle wasting, alopecia, seborrhea, and urinary tract infection. ACTH stimulation and dexamethasone suppression testing confirmed hyperadrenocorticism. On ultrasonography, a right adrenal gland mass was identified. A unilateral adrenalectomy was performed and impression smears of the mass prepared for cytologic examination (**19a, b**; Leishman's, ×40 and ×100 oil, respectively). The mass was submitted for histologic evaluation.

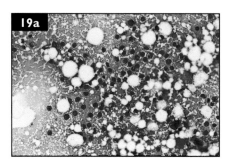
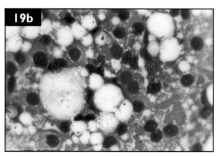

1 Describe the cytologic features of the nucleated cells.
2 What is the likely origin/type of these cells?
3 Based on this group of cells, what diagnosis would you make in this case?

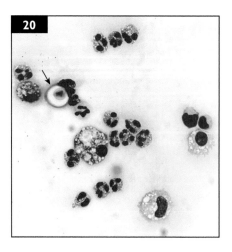

CASE 20 A 5-year-old German Shorthaired Pointer was presented with a history of acute cervical hyperesthesia and neurologic deficits on the forelimbs. The dog was hospitalized and despite cage rest and analgesic therapy it deteriorated overnight, becoming nonambulatory and assuming sternal recumbency. MRI of the cervical and thoracic spine showed a diffuse intramedullary hyperintensity affecting the cervical and thoracic regions. CSF was collected from the cisterna magna. A smear of the CSF is shown (**20**; Wright–Giemsa, ×50 oil).

1 Describe the findings seen in the photomicrograph.
2 What is your interpretation based on these cytologic findings?

CASE 21 A cat presented with pyrexia, pneumonia, and dyspnea. Pleural fluid was obtained and smears made from sediment from the fluid are shown (**21a, b**; Wright–Giemsa, ×50 oil and ×100 oil, respectively). Similar findings were also obtained from a bronchoalveolar lavage.

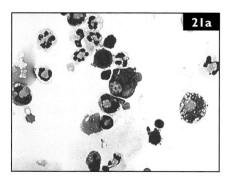 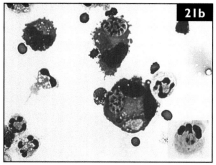

1 Identify the etiologic agent in this exudative effusion, with precise reference to the exact stage of its life cycle as seen in the photomicrographs.
2 What other laboratory tests would you like to use to support your cytologic suspicion?
3 Given the following laboratory results, what can you determine about the kinetics of *Toxoplasma gondii* from these values: IgM – ELISA ~1:256; IgG – ELISA ~1:64?
4 Toxoplasmosis is a potential zoonotic risk. Are cat owners and veterinarians at significantly higher risk than the general population of acquiring *T. gondii* infection?
5 Are seropositive cats a risk for pregnant women or immunocompromised individuals?

CASE 22 Quality assurance programs are required to monitor, evaluate, and improve laboratory performances. Guidelines for quality assurance programs in veterinary cytology have been provided by the American Society for Veterinary Clinical Pathology Committee on Quality Assurance and Laboratory Standards.

1 What are the principles of quality assurance in veterinary cytology, and how can diagnostic accuracy be determined in veterinary cytology?

CASE 23 An FNA is collected with ultrasound guidance from a hypoechoic lesion within the pancreas. Smears of the aspirate are shown (**23a, b**; Wright–Giemsa, ×10 and ×100 oil, respectively).

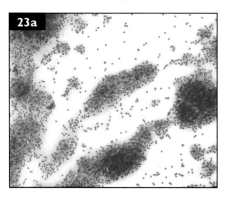

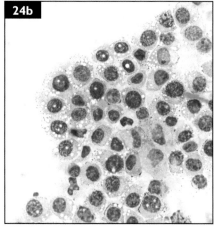

1 Describe the cells shown in the photomicrographs.
2 What is your interpretation of these findings?

CASE 24 A 2-year-old mixed-breed dog presented with a history of a cauliflower-like mass on the dorsal side of the penis (**24a**). An FNA from the mass was obtained. A smear of the aspirate is shown (**24b**; Wright–Giemsa, ×50 oil).

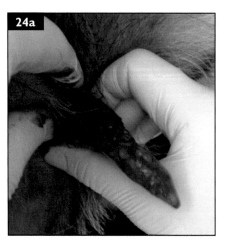

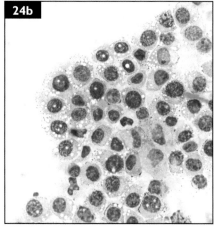

1 Describe the cells shown in the photomicrograph.
2 What is your interpretation of these cytologic findings?

CASE 25 An FNA is collected from a feline lymph node. Smears of the aspirate are shown (**25a–c; a, b**, May–Grünwald–Giemsa, ×40 and ×100 oil, respectively; **c**, Ziehl–Neelsen, ×100 oil).

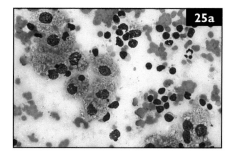

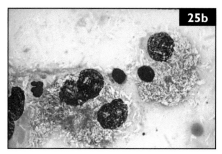

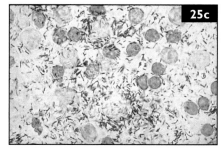

1 Describe the cells represented in the smears.
2 What is your interpretation, and what are the differential diagnoses?

CASE 26 A 1-year-old neutered male DSH cat presented with a history of lethargy and anorexia. Clinical examination revealed icteric mucous membranes. Abnormal biochemistry findings included: ALT = 114 U/l (RI = 32–87 U/l); GGT = 14.3 (RI = 0.1–0.6 U/l): total bilirubin = 73 μmol/l (RI = 2.4–4.4 μmol/l); TP = 95 g/l (RI = 63–78 g/l); albumin = 28 g/l (RI = 30–40 g/l); globulin = 67 g/dl (RI = 30–45 g/l). A smear from an FNA of the liver is shown (**26**; May–Grünwald–Giemsa, ×100 oil).

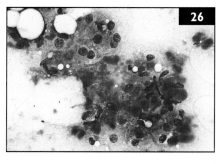

1 Describe the cytologic findings, and give your cytologic interpretation.
2 What additional tests might be useful in order to confirm the diagnosis?

13

CASE 27 An 8-year-old dog presented with clinical signs of pyrexia and a marked toxic leukogram with a degenerative left shift. Bronchoalveolar lavage was performed. Smears from the lavage wash are shown (**27a–c**; **a**, **b**, Wright–Giemsa, ×50 oil; **c**, Wright–Giemsa, ×100 oil).

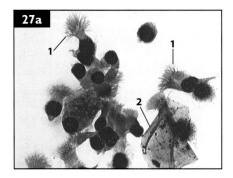

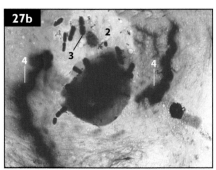

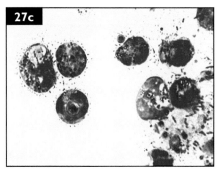

1 Identify the cells or structures labeled 1, 2, 3, and 4 in **27a** and **27b**, and state their significance in the context of a bronchoalveolar lavage.
2 Interpret the pathologic process seen in **27c**.
3 How do you know that the bacteria present in this wash are likely to be significant?

4 Are eosinophils more or less effective at phagocytosing and killing bacteria than neutrophils?

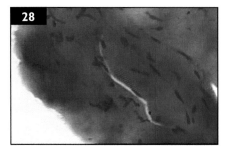

CASE 28 An FNA is collected from a firm mass on the neck of a 7-year-old Welsh cob gelding. A smear of the aspirate is shown (**28**; Wright–Giemsa, ×100 oil).

1 Describe the structure shown in the smear.
2 What is your interpretation?
3 What are your differential diagnoses?

CASE 29 A 13-year-old neutered male Fox Terrier presented with a history of vomiting and abdominal pain. On clinical examination the dog was in poor body condition and had icteric mucous membranes. Abnormal hematology findings included: WBCs = 12.99 × 10^9/l (RI = 5.45–12.98 × 10^{09}/l); monocytes = 1.03 × 10^9/l (RI = 0.18–0.79 × 10^9/l). Neutrophils showed signs of left shift and toxic changes. Abnormal biochemistry findings included: AST = 112 U/l (RI = 15–35 U/l); ALT = 1,487 (RI = 32–87 U/l): ALP= 7,235 (RI = 19–70 U/l): GGT= 135.4 (RI = 0.1–0.6 U/l); total bilirubin = 117.4 µmol/l (RI = 2.4–4.4 µmol/l); cholesterol = 11.8 mmol/l (RI = 4.03–9.54 mmol/l); C reactive protein = 623.1 mg/l (RI = 0.1–2.2 mg/l); haptoglobin = 243 g/l (RI = 10–960 g/l). A smear from an FNA of the liver is shown (**29**; May–Grünwald–Giemsa, ×100 oil).

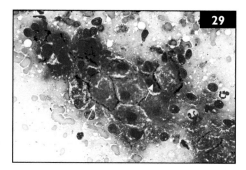

1 What is the most important feature in this liver aspirate?
2 Based on all these findings, what is the most likely cause for this condition?

CASE 30 A 3-year-old neutered male dog was presented for a golf ball sized subcutaneous nodule on the neck that ruptured and was drained 4 weeks previously. The dog was treated with amoxicillin and steroids at that time, with a presumptive diagnosis of abscess formation. Multiple ulcerated cutaneous masses developed over the intervening weeks. An FNA was obtained from one of the new developing lesions. A smear of the aspirate is shown (**30**; Wright–Giemsa, ×100 oil).

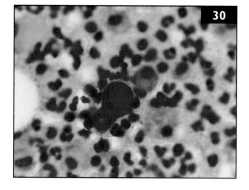

1 Identify the organism.
2 What is the primary morphologic finding used to identify this organism?

CASE 31 You have been treating a 5-year-old Newfoundland with otitis externa for several weeks with a topical ear ointment. Because of a poor clinical response you make a few cytologic smears from the copious, dark-brown exudate (sweet odor) (**31a, b;** Wright–Giemsa, ×10 and ×100 oil, respectively).

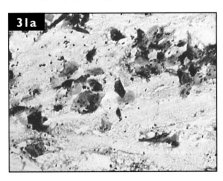 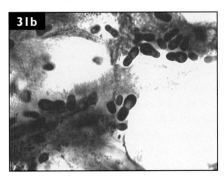

1 Describe your findings.
2 How do you decide whether yeasts are significant or not?
3 By what proposed theories does *Malassezia* cause otitis?
4 What special stains can be used to demonstrate *Malassezia*, and what are the staining characteristics with these stains?

CASE 32 An FNA was collected from a firm, demarcated, cutaneous, mobile skin mass in a dog. Smears of the aspirate are shown (**32a, b;** Wright–Giemsa, ×50 oil and ×100 oil, respectively).

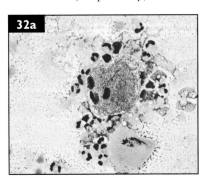 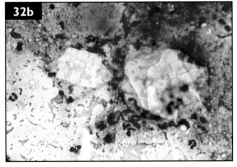

1 What processes are indicated in the photomicrographs?
2 What is your final interpretation?

CASE 33 A spongy mass is found on the bone lateral and caudal to the eye in a 9-year-old horse from a riding stable. An FNA is collected (**33a**). A smear from the aspirate is shown (**33b**; Wright–Giemsa, ×100 oil).

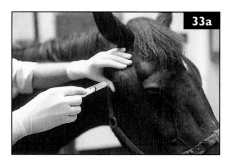
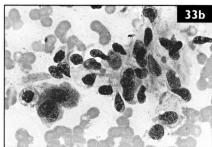

1 What cells are present?
2 What is your interpretation?

CASE 34 A 10-year-old entire male Yorkshire Terrier was presented for annual vaccination. Clinical examination revealed a firm fixed mass, 1 cm in diameter, located below the anus in the 6 o'clock position. Smears from an FNA of the mass are shown (**34a, b**; both May–Grünwald–Giemsa, ×40).

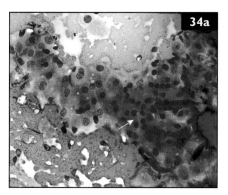
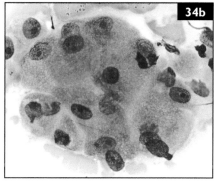

1 Describe the cytologic findings of these photomicrographs.
2 What is your interpretation?

CASE 35 An 8-year-old entire female Boxer was referred for investigation of occasional coughing episodes and for the presence of a large deep mass in the ventral region of the neck, lateral to the trachea. An aspirate was collected from the mass. Smears of the aspirate are shown (35a, b; May–Grünwald–Giemsa, ×40 and ×100 oil, respectively).

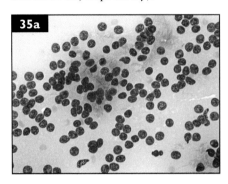

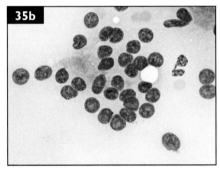

1 Describe the cytologic features seen in the photomicrographs, and provide a general description.
2 What is your interpretation, and what further investigations would you recommend?

CASE 36 A Friesian cow has swollen eyelids, with marked blepharospasm and an ocular discharge (36a). An FNA is collected. A smear of the aspirate is shown (36b; Wright–Giemsa, ×100 oil).

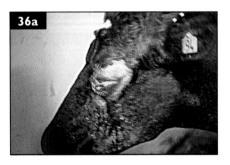

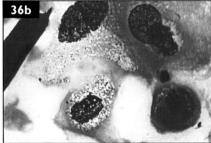

1 What cells are present?
2 What is the cytologic interpretation?

CASE 37 A skin scrape is collected from a crusting variably alopecic lesion on the head of a dog. The sample is cleared with diluted alkali (10% potassium hydroxide) then photographed after 15 minutes (**37a, b**; unstained, ×10 and ×100 oil, respectively).

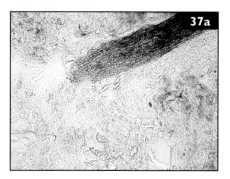 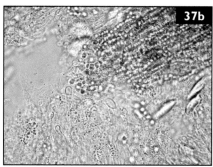

1 Describe the features shown.
2 What is your interpretation of these findings?

CASE 38 A 3-year-old Thoroughbred racehorse is referred for investigation of poor performance. A bronchoalveolar lavage specimen is collected as part of the work up. Smears of the lavage fluid are shown (**38a, b**; Papanicolaou, ×50 oil and ×100 oil, respectively).

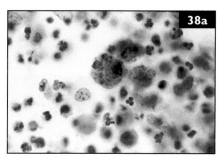 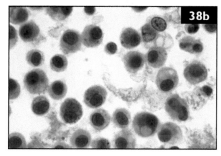

1 What cell types are present in the photomicrographs?
2 What differences do you notice in the siderophages shown in the photomicrographs?
3 What is your interpretation of the cytologic findings?

19

CASE 39 An adult entire female boxer presented with a distinct but irregular mass within a mammary gland. Aspiration of the mass was performed. Smears of the aspirate are shown (**39a, b**; Wright–Giemsa, ×20 and ×100 oil, respectively).

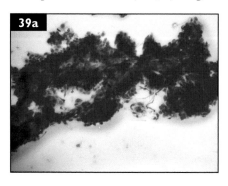
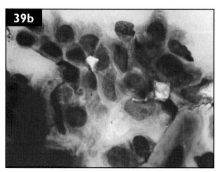

1 Describe the features shown in the photomicrographs.
2 What is your interpretation of these findings?

CASE 40 An aged Labrador Retriever has a firm painless mass on its gum (**40a**). An FNA is collected. A smear of the aspirate is shown (**40b**; Wright–Giemsa, ×100 oil).

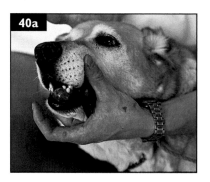
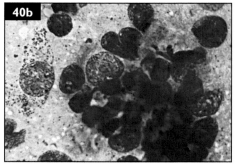

1 What cells are present?
2 What is your interpretation?

CASE 41 An 11-year-old entire male German Wirehaired Pointer presented with a mass on the lateral right hock. The mass was firm, nonpainful, and 1 cm in diameter. Smears of an FNA of the mass are shown (41a, b; May–Grünwald–Giemsa, ×20 and ×100 oil, respectively).

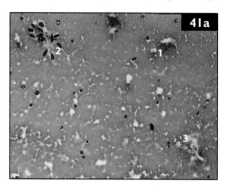
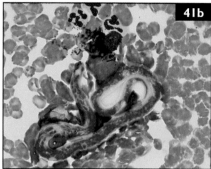

1 Describe the cytologic findings, and give your cytologic interpretation.
2 What additional tests might be useful to confirm the diagnosis?

CASE 42 A 1-year-old spayed female mongrel dog presented for evaluation of a 5 cm subcutaneous mass in the interscapular region. The dog was recently spayed. An FNA was obtained. Smears of the aspirate are shown (42a, b; May–Grünwald–Giemsa, ×40 and ×100 oil, respectively).

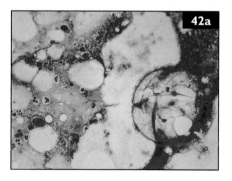
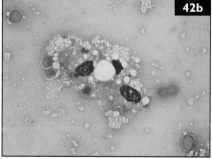

1 Identify the cell population present in the smear, and describe the most relevant characteristics.
2 What is your final interpretation?

CASE 43 A 15-month-old entire male English Springer Spaniel presented with a chronic, worsening productive cough. The dog had shown no response to a 1-week course of doxycycline and it had recently become anorexic. On clinical examination the dog was slightly pyrexic. Radiographs of the thorax revealed a bronchopneumonia and endoscopy a severe tonsillitis, laryngitis, and tracheitis. Smears of some expectorated material are shown (**43a, b**; modified Wright's, ×10 and ×100 respectively).

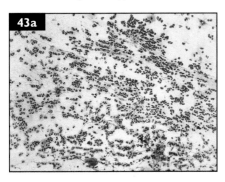 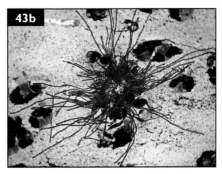

1 Describe the features illustrated.
2 What is your interpretation of these findings?
3 What other conditions is this organism associated with?

CASE 44 A smear from an FNA collected from a submandibular lymph node of a 13-year-old female crossbred dog is shown (**44**; Wright–Giemsa, ×50 oil).

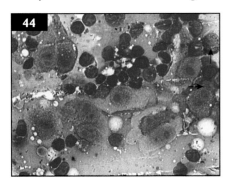

1 Describe the cells seen in the smear. What is your interpretation?
2 Based on the cytologic features of the metastatic cells, indicate the most likely differential diagnosis.
3 Which special stains could you use to confirm your diagnosis?
4 Which tumors tend to metastasize to regional lymph nodes: carcinomas or sarcomas?

CASE 45 A 3-year-old spayed female Cavalier King Charles Spaniel presented with a history of coughing and dyspnea. Thoracic radiography revealed a generalized bronchointerstitial pattern. A bronchoalveolar lavage (BAL) sample was taken and submitted for analysis. Smears of the sample are shown (**45a, b**; Wright–Giemsa, ×10 and ×50 oil, respectively).

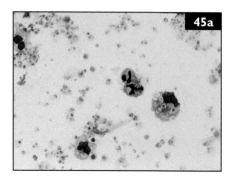
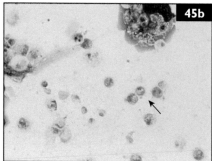

1 Which types of inflammatory cells can be seen in this BAL sample?
2 What are the structures indicated by the arrow in **45b**?

CASE 46 An ultrasound-guided FNA was collected from an irregular hypoechoic lesion within the pancreas of a dog. Smears of the aspirate are shown (**46a, b**; Wright–Giemsa, ×20 and ×100 oil, respectively).

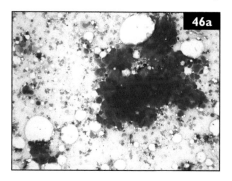
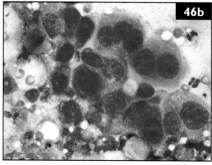

1 Describe the features shown in the photomicrographs.
2 What is your interpretation of these findings?

23

CASE 47 A 16-week-old Shih Tzu presented with mucoid diarrhea. The puppy was outwardly well and had a good appetite. A zinc sulfate fecal float (×40) was made (47a). A saline mount (×40) was made for comparison (47b).

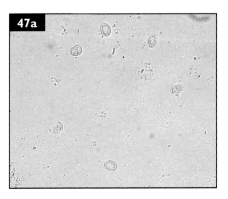
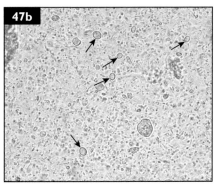

1 What are these organisms?
2 Describe how and where to look on the zinc sulfate fecal float to find the cysts.
3 Are yeast cells larger or smaller than these cysts? Do they float?

CASE 48 A 6-year-old female Schnauzer presented with polyuria/polydipsia and frequent nocturnal urination. Physical examination revealed that the dog was bright and alert, slightly overweight, and had a distended abdomen. An enlarged liver was evident on abdominal palpation. The rest of the physical examination

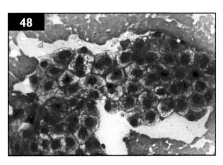

was within normal limits. Abnormal biochemistry values were as follows: AST = 253 U/l (RI = 14–38 U/l); ALT = 450 U/l (RI = 10–71 U/l); ALP = 2,300 U/l (RI = 4–110 U/l); glucose = 7.78 mmol/l (RI = 4.4–7.0 mmol/l); bilirubin = 1.7 µmol/l (RI = 0–6.8 µmol/l). An FNA of the liver was obtained. A smear of the aspirate is shown (48; Wright–Giemsa, ×20).

1 Describe the cytologic features seen in the FNA, and give an interpretation.
2 Briefly discuss the biochemical profile. How does it support your cytologic findings?
3 Discuss additional diagnostic tests to confirm the underlying disease process.

CASE 49 An 11-year-old male Rottweiler was presented with a history of weakness, lethargy, and lameness. A bone marrow FNA was collected. Smears of the aspirate are shown (**49a, b**; May–Grünwald–Giemsa, ×40 and ×100 oil, respectively).

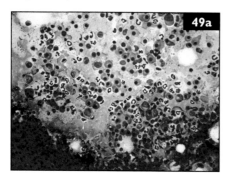
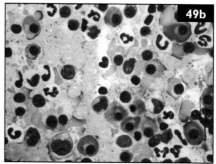

1 Describe the cells present in the smear, and provide an overall interpretation.
2 What is your final interpretation, and what additional work up is needed to confirm the hypothesis?

CASE 50 A 4-year-old neutered male Shi-Tzu was referred for stranguria, pollakiuria, and hematuria. The dog was previously treated with antibiotics for suspected cystitis. Abdominal radiographs revealed a single radiodense urolith in the bladder; no nephroliths or uretroliths were found. Urinalysis was performed and revealed: USG = 1.046 (RI = 1.020–1.045); pH = 5.0 (RI = 5.0–7.0). Urine dipstick was positive for protein (++) and blood (++++). Urine sediment examination identified large numbers of RBCs and crystals (**50a**; unstained urine sediment, ×40), together with moderate numbers of leukocytes and transitional epithelial cells.

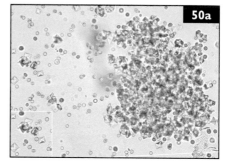

1 What crystals are shown in the photomicrograph?
2 At what pH range do these crystals form?
3 How can the hematuria be explained?

25

CASE 51 An 8-year-old broodmare (three previous foals) presents with a history of repeated uterine infections that had been treated with antibiotics. A uterine washing is collected to determine the mare's status. Smears of the wash are shown (**51a, b**; Papanicolaou, ×50 oil and ×100 oil, respectively).

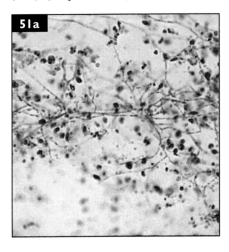
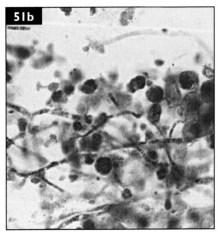

1 Describe the features shown.
2 What is your interpretation of these findings?
3 What is the significance of these findings?

CASE 52 A 12-year old spayed female DLH cat presented for decreased activity, weight loss, and difficulty breathing. On physical examination, the cat was dyspneic and pyrexic. Radiographs revealed myriad, multifocal, small, ill-defined opacities throughout the lung fields. A cytocentrifuged preparation of bronchoalveolar lavage fluid is shown (**52**; Wright–Giemsa, ×100 oil).

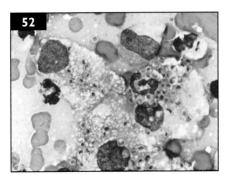

1 Identify the organism.
2 What are the common routes of infection?

CASE 53 A 5-year-old Boxer presented with acute onset of unilateral epistaxis. The dog appeared underweight and physical examination revealed generalized lymphadenopathy. An FNA was obtained from the left popliteal lymph node. Smears of the aspirate are shown (53a, b; Wright–Giemsa, ×50 oil and ×100 oil, respectively).

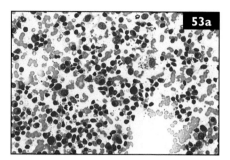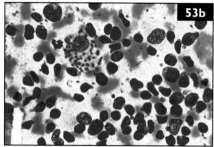

1 Describe the main changes present in 53a? The large cell in the center of 53b represents a mononuclear phagocyte. Describe the organisms within the cytoplasm. What is your interpretation?
2 Laboratory investigation revealed nonregenerative anemia, hyperglobulinemia characterized by polyclonal gammopathy, and mild renal azotemia. A coagulation panel was unremarkable. How can the epistaxis be explained?

CASE 54 A 7-year-old spayed female Labrador Retriever presented with a history of acute crusting/cracking to dorsal surface of the nose. Some mild nose leather (the naked skin around a cat's nostrils) graying (depigmentation) was present as well. Clinical signs improved but did not resolve with a topical immunosuppressant. The dog developed scaling with thickening of the skin along the periocular/lid margins. A skin biopsy of an early developing pustular lesion and an aspirate of the contents of a larger pustule were obtained. A smear of the aspirate is shown (54a; Wright–Giemsa, ×40).

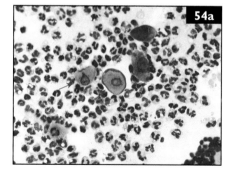

1 Identify the structures indicated by the arrow.
2 List two differentials for this finding.

CASE 55 Abdominocentesis was performed on a cat with an inflammatory leukogram and a toxic left shift (**55a**). Biochemistry revealed moderately increased ALP and ALT and mild azotemia. Fluid analysis: TP = 33.9 g/l; albumin = 14.1 g/l; globulin = 19.8 g/l; albumin:globulin ratio = 0.7; SG = 1.028; NCC = 150.9 × 10^9/l; RBCs = 0.04 × 10^{12}/l. A smear of the fluid is shown (**55b**; Wright–Giemsa, ×100 oil).

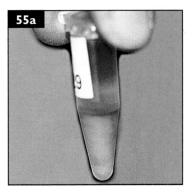
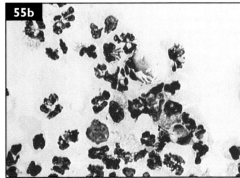

1 Interpret the fluid specimen using the laboratory data and the photomicrograph.
2 In view of the fact that the sample contained a pleomorphic bacterial population, including rods, cocci, and filamentous bacteria, select two further laboratory tests that you would like to run or be sent to a referral laboratory.
3 What are the most common bacteria isolated from pyothorax and septic peritonitis?

CASE 56 A weanling foal presented with pyrexia, moderate mucopurulent nasal discharge and wheezes, and crackles on thoracic auscultation. A tracheal washing was collected. A smear of the wash is shown (**56a**; Sano's modification of Pollack's Trichrome, ×50 oil).

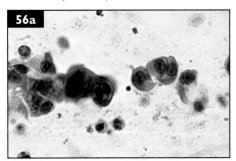

1 What are the cells shown in the photomicrograph?
2 What is the significance of this finding?

CASE 57 A 3-year-old spayed female DSH cat presented 3 weeks post parturition with a history of respiratory distress. On physical examination, the cat exhibited tachypnea, tachycardia, and pyrexia. Abdominal palpation revealed a large caudal intra-abdominal mass. An aspirate of the abdominal mass was submitted for cytology (57a, b; Wright–Giemsa, ×60 and ×100 oil, respectively).

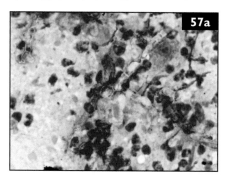
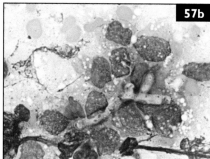

1 What is your cytologic interpretation?
2 List possible differentials for this organism.

CASE 58 An 11-year-old spayed female Yorkshire Terrier was referred for bilateral enlargement of the submandibular area. An FNA from the area was collected. Smears of the aspirate are shown (58a, b; Wright–Giemsa, ×10 and ×50 oil, respectively).

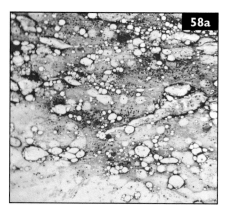
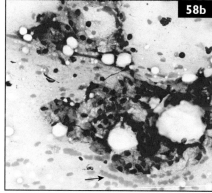

1 What cell types are shown in the photomicrographs?
2 Photomicrograph 58b shows a linear arrangement of the erythrocytes (indicated by the arrow), known as 'wind-rowing'. What is the cause of this?

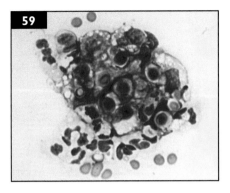

CASE 59 A 3-year-old neutered male DSH cat presents with inspiratory dyspnea and severe nasal congestion of 4 months' duration. The cat has lost weight and shown partial anorexia in the last few weeks. Physical examination reveals approximately 10% dehydration, hyperthermia (39.8°C [103.6°F]), unilateral mucosanguineous nasal discharge, and ipsilateral submandibular lymph node enlargement. The referring veterinarian had administered enrofloxacin, doxycycline, and amoxicillin/clavulanic acid successively and no improvement was noted. Vaccinations are up-to-date and the cat is free roaming. A smear of the nasal discharge is shown (59; Wright's, ×100 oil).

1 What is your interpretation based on cytologic observation?
2 What other diagnostic tests can be performed to support this diagnosis?

CASE 60 An 8-year-old spayed female DSH cat presented with a 2-week history of intermittent vomiting. There was an acute onset of lethargy and anorexia. Significant findings on physical examination included icterus and severe hepatomegaly. CBC findings

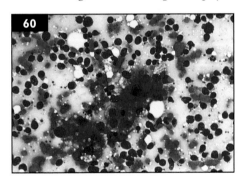

included moderate, nonregenerative anaemia (PCV = 0.23 l/l). Abnormal biochemistry findings were: ALT = 360 U/l (RI = 10–80 U/l); ALP = 120 U/L (RI = 2–43 U/l); bilirubin = 55 μmol/l (RI = 0–3.4 μmol/l). An FNA of the liver was obtained. A smear of the aspirate is shown (60; Wright–Giemsa, ×25).

1 Describe the cytologic findings, and give your cytologic interpretation.
2 Discuss the condition.

CASE 61 Identify the exogenous and possible foreign body material in the photomicrograph (**61**; Wright–Giemsa, ×100 oil).

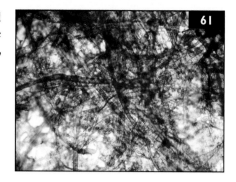

CASE 62 A 9-year-old spayed female DSH cat was presented with a submandibular swelling. Fine needle aspiration of cervical lymph nodes was performed. A smear of the aspirate is shown (**62**; May–Grünwald–Giemsa, ×100 oil).

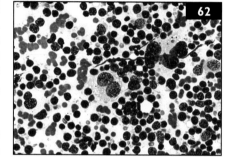

1 Identify the main cell populations present in the smear, and describe the most relevant characteristics.
2 What is your interpretation?

CASE 63 A 14-year-old carriage horse in New York City presented with a history of chronic coughing. A tracheal washing was collected and a smear prepared (**63**; Alcian Blue–PAS overlaid on Papanicolaou, ×40).

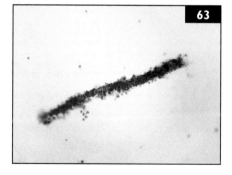

1 What is the structure shown in the photomicrograph?
2 What is its significance?

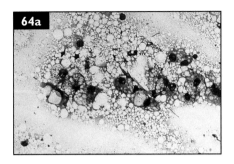

64a

CASE 64 A 6-year-old spayed female DSH cat presented for chronic weight loss and a recent history of vomiting and severe lethargy. Physical examination revealed pale, icteric mucous membranes. The temperature was 38°C (100.4°F) and pulse and respiration rates were slightly increased. Abdominal palpation and radiographs revealed diffuse hepatomegaly. Examination of a peripheral blood smear indicated RBC shape abnormalities including severe acanthocytosis. Abnormal biochemistry values were: AST = 150 U/l (RI = 2–36 U/l); ALT = 350 U/l (RI = 6–80 U/l); ALP = 135 U/l (RI = 2–43 U/l); bilirubin = 68 µmol/l (RI = 0–3.4 µmol/l). An FNA of the liver was obtained. A smear of the aspirate is shown (64a; Wright–Giemsa, ×25).

1 Explain the abnormal RBC shape and the biochemistry abnormalities.
2 Describe the cytologic findings and give your cytologic interpretation.
3 List the differentials for your diagnosis.

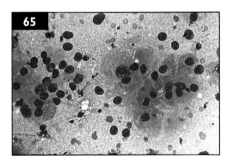

65

CASE 65 A 10-year-old neutered male Shetland Sheepdog presented with a history of diarrhea, vomiting, anorexia, and lethargy of 3 days' duration. Physical examination findings included weight loss; a cranial abdominal mass was detected on abdominal palpation. Thoracic radiographs were normal. Abdominal radiographs revealed an enlarged liver that displaced the stomach and intestines and obstructed the pyloric outflow of the stomach. Ultrasound evaluation of the abdomen showed diffuse involvement of the entire liver. CBC findings included moderate anemia, leukopenia, and thrombocytopenia. The biochemistry profile showed: AST = 8,480 U/l (RI = 14–38 U/l); ALT = 10,900 U/l (RI = 10–71 U/l); ALP = 1,476 U/l (RI = 4–110 U/l); bilirubin = 202 µmol/l (RI = 0–6.8 µmol/l); BUN = 1.4 mmol/l (RI = 2.1–9.4 mmol/l); TP = 44 g/l (RI = 56–75 g/l). A smear from an FNA of the liver is shown (65; Wright–Giemsa, ×25).

1 Describe the cytologic findings, and give your cytologic interpretation.
2 Discuss the various forms of this disease seen in the dog.
3 Discuss the prognosis for this patient.

CASE 66 A 6-year-old neutered male Rottweiler presented with a history of stiffness, lethargy, and slight bilateral stifle joint effusions. No cranial drawer sign was present. Synovial fluid was collected from both stifle joints; the fluid from both joints contained similar features (**66a, b**; Wright Giemsa, ×50 oil and ×100 oil, respectively). Analysis of the synovial fluid revealed: RBCs = <10 × 10^{12}/l; NCC = 3.2 × 10^9/l; TP = 40 g/l; mucin clot test – normal; viscosity – normal.

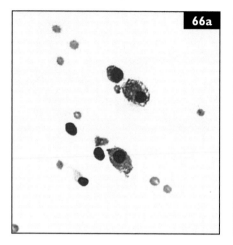

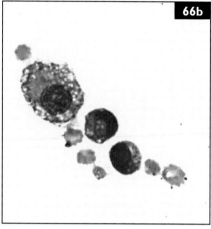

1 Describe the cell types and features illustrated in the two photomicrographs.
2 What is your interpretation of this case, and what are your comments?

CASE 67 A 9-year-old entire male German Shepherd Dog was presented for restaging of an unresectable cutaneous mast cell tumor, previously treated with chemotherapy and radiotherapy. Abdominal ultrasound revealed slight liver enlargement and diffuse increased echogenicity. An FNA was collected and submitted for analysis. A smear of the aspirate is shown (**67**; Wright–Giemsa, ×100 oil).

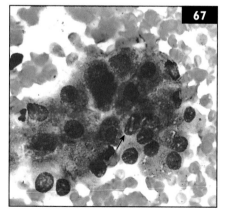

1 What is the structure indicated by the arrow?

CASE 68 A 6-year-old neutered male Labrador Retriever presented with a history of nonweight bearing lameness of the right forelimb after jumping off a bed. Radiographs revealed a lytic-proliferative bone lesion of the distal right humerus. Four trephine biopsies were obtained via a craniolateral surgical approach. Roll preparations were submitted for cytologic evaluation (**68a, b**; both Wright–Giemsa, ×50 oil).

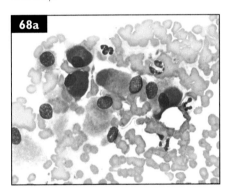
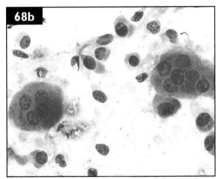

1 What is the predominant cell type in photomicrograph **68a**?
2 What are the large multinucleated cells in photomicrograph **68b**?
3 What is your most likely diagnosis?
4 What additional cytochemical stain could be performed to help assess the cell type of origin?

CASE 69 A 12-year-old neutered male Jack Russell Terrier was referred for an enlarged and painful abdomen. Clinical examination revealed a palpable mass in the cranial abdomen. Hematologic, biochemical, and urinary findings were unremarkable. Abdominal ultrasound confirmed the presence of a mass, which was localized to the right lobe of the liver. A smear from an FNA of the liver is shown (**69**; May–Grünwald–Giemsa, ×100 oil).

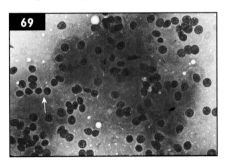

1 Describe the cytologic findings, and give your cytologic interpretation.
2 What additional tests might be useful in order to confirm the diagnosis?

CASE 70 A 7-year-old half-bred mare was unthrifty and eating poorly. A sample of peritoneal fluid was yellow, mildly turbid, and had an NCC of 27 ×10⁹/l and a TP of 47 g/l. A cytospun smear of the fluid was made (**70a**; Wright–Giemsa, ×100 oil). On rectal examination a spherical mass was palpated in mid-abdomen. Fluid from the mass was aspirated under ultrasound guidance. A smear from the fluid is shown (**70b**; Wright–Giemsa, ×100 oil).

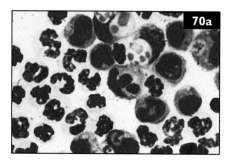
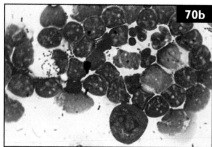

1 What type of fluid (fluid classification) is present in the abdomen?
2 What are the cells shown in **70a**?
3 What are the cells shown in **70b**?
4 What is your interpretation?

CASE 71 Pleural fluid is collected from a 1-year-old cat with pleural effusion. Fluid analysis: TP = 40.9 g/l; albumin = 23.2 g/l; globulin = 17.7 g/l; albumin:globulin ratio = 1.3; SG = 1.030; NCC = 17.76 × 10⁹/l; RBCs = 0.32 × 10¹²/l. A smear of the fluid is shown (**71**; Wright–Giemsa, ×100 oil).

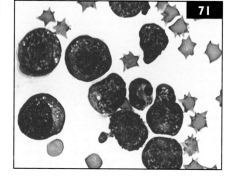

1 Review the laboratory data and photomicrograph, and give an appropriate interpretation.
2 Given the young age of this cat and the anatomic location of the lymphoma, what other laboratory data would you like to obtain that may affect the prognosis of this patient?

CASE 72 An 18-month-old German Shepherd Dog-cross presented with a dome-shaped mass of approximately 3 cm diameter in the area of the right distal antebrachium, near the elbow joint. Gritty chalky material with a cheesy consistency was aspirated. A smear of the aspirate is shown (72a; Wright–Giemsa, ×100 oil).

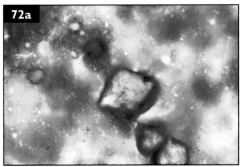

1 What can be seen in the smear?
2 What is your interpretation?

CASE 73 A 4-year-old spayed female dog presented for a chronic draining skin lesion located on the flank. A CBC and chemistry profile revealed a mature neutrophilia and monocytosis with hyperglobulinemia. The lesion was not responsive to broad-spectrum antibiotics. An FNA of the lesion was obtained. Smears of the aspirate are shown (73a, b; both Wright–Giemsa, ×60).

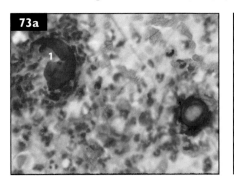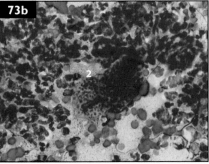

1 Identify the organism.
2 Identify the structures labeled 1 and 2.
3 What are the two most common organ systems affected by this disease in the dog?

CASE 74 A 5-year-old spayed female Labrador Retriever presented for a 3–4-week history of limping on the right forelimb, which was initially attributed to a history of a mink bite. Recently, the lameness had worsened despite treatment with analgesics. On physical examination, the right prescapular lymph node was moderately enlarged and there was a large 10 cm × 7 cm, nonpainful mass in the right axillary region accompanied by a firm swelling of the left elbow with decreased range of motion. Biopsies for histopathology were collected from sources identified on physical examination. CT revealed that the dog had a single kidney, which was characterized by multiple nodular lesions. A cytology sample was collected. Smears of the sample are shown (**74a, b**; Wright–Giemsa, ×20 and ×50 oil, respectively).

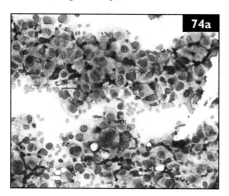 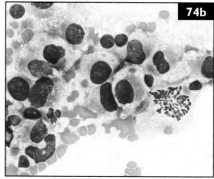

1 Based on these photomicrographs, describe the cells. Are they consistent with normal renal tissue?
2 What is the most likely cytologic diagnosis?
3 What tests could be performed to confirm this diagnosis?

CASE 75 A 5-year-old spayed female DSH cat presented with a history of vomiting, anorexia, diarrhea, and depression. Abdominal ultrasound identified an intestinal mass, which was aspirated. A smear of the aspirate is shown (**75**; May–Grünwald–Giemsa, ×100 oil).

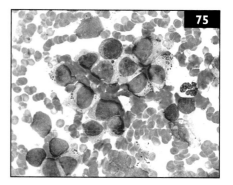

1 Describe the cell population in the photomicrograph.
2 What is your interpretation?

CASE 76 A Friesian cow (**76a**) presented because it was thin and was scouring. A hemispherical mass on its flank was aspirated. A smear of the aspirate is shown (**76b**; Wright–Giemsa, ×100 oil).

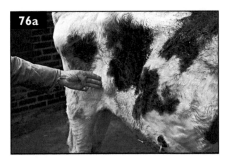 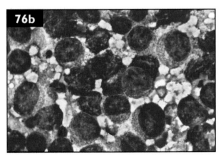

1 What cells are present?
2 What is your interpretation?

CASE 77 An 8-year-old Thoroughbred-cross gelding presented with suspected polyuria and polydipsia. A urine sample was collected. Smears made from the urine sediment are shown (**77a, b**; Wright–Giemsa, ×50 oil and ×100 oil, respectively).

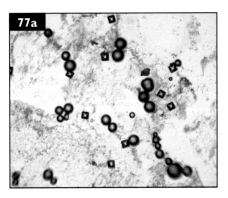 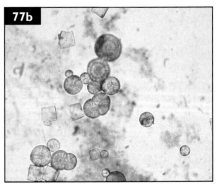

1 What are the structures shown in the smears?
2 What is the significance of these findings?
3 What is your interpretation?

CASE 78 A 3.5-year-old entire male Golden Retriever presented with a well-circumscribed, moderately firm, frontal, subcutaneous mass, 4 cm in diameter that had been noted a few weeks previously by its owner. Cranial radiographs revealed a well-circumscribed mass associated with mild osteolysis and bony proliferation in the left frontal sinus. When aspirated, a blood-tinged viscous material was obtained. Photomicrographs at low-power and high-power magnification illustrate the cytologic appearance of this tumor (78a–c; Wright's, ×10, ×100 oil, and ×100 oil, respectively).

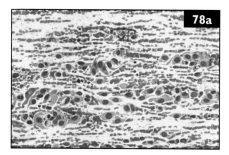

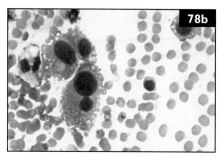

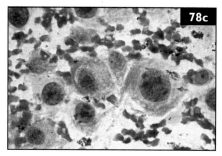

1 What are your differential diagnoses?

CASE 79 A 14-year-old spayed female DSH cat was presented with a history of ptyalism and dysorexia. Clinical examination revealed a mass localized in the basal part of the tongue and hypertrophy of the left retromandibular lymph node. A smear from an FNA of the lymph node is shown (79; May–Grünwald–Giemsa, ×40).

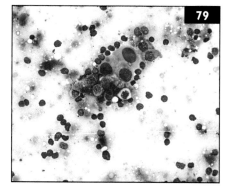

1 Describe the cytologic findings, and give your cytologic interpretation.

39

CASE 80 A 12-year-old spayed female Border Collie presented for decreased interest in normal activities and decreased exercise tolerance. The owners had noted an increased respiratory rate and possibly some difficulty with defecation. Abdominal ultrasound revealed multiple, complex cavitated liver masses, a large mass at the head of the spleen, and enlarged intra-abdominal lymph nodes. A CBC showed an inflammatory leukogram, a moderate regenerative anemia, and a mild thrombocytopenia. Ultrasound-guided aspiration of the liver masses were performed and smears were submitted for cytology (**80a, b**; Wright–Giemsa, ×20 and ×50 oil, respectively).

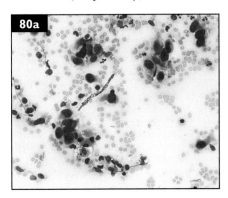
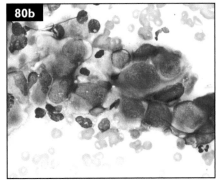

1 The cells seen in the photomicrographs are most consistent with what general cell lineage?
2 Given the tissue distribution of the lesions, the clinical history, and the hematologic data, what is the most likely specific neoplasm in this dog?

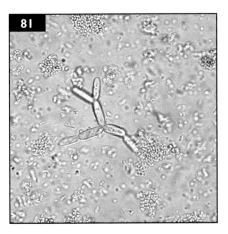

CASE 81 A 6-year-old neutered male mixed-breed dog presented for routine vaccinations. A fecal flotation sample had many of these large, symmetrical, sausage-shaped organisms (**81**; unstained zinc sulfate flotation sample, ×40).

1 Is this a parasite?
2 What is it?

CASE 82 Hemorrhagic pleural fluid (**82a**) was aspirated from a 9-year-old Doberman Pinscher that presented with clinical signs of dyspnea and mild pallor. Smears of the fluid are shown (**82b, c**; both Wright–Giemsa, ×100 oil).

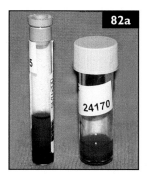

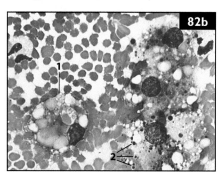

1 Identify the structures/cells labeled 1, 2, 3, and 4, and state their significance.
2 Which of the findings indicate chronic hemorrhage?
3 Which special stain would you request to confirm that hemosiderin (labeled 2) from blood breakdown pigment is present and contains iron?

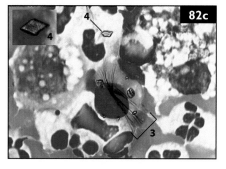

4 List three common causes of hemorrhagic effusions and the relevant laboratory tests you can use in the investigation of the causes of hemorrhagic effusions.

CASE 83 An FNA is collected from a cystic mass on the lumbar area of a 6-year-old entire male Border Collie. A smear of the aspirate is shown (**83**; Wright–Giemsa, ×50 oil).

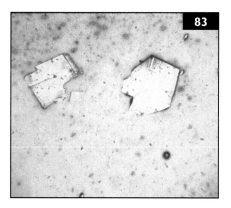

1 Describe the cytologic findings.
2 What is the significance of these findings?
3 What is your cytologic interpretation, and what are your comments?

41

CASE 84 A bone marrow aspirate was performed on a 10-year-old spayed female Whippet with a history of moderate thrombocytopenia ($85 \times 10^9/l$ [RI = 180–$550 \times 10^9/l$]) and marked hyperglobulinemia (113 g/l [RI = 15–60 g/l]), with an oligoclonal pattern of the β_2-globulins. Smears of the aspirate are shown (84a, b; both Modified Wright's, ×50 oil)?

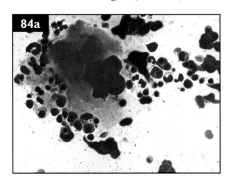
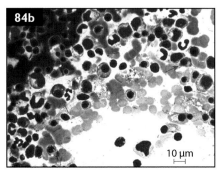

1 What is the very large cell present in 84a?
2 What are the small cells indicated by the arrows in 84b?
3 What diseases can cause an increase in these cells in the bone marrow?

CASE 85 A 4-year-old male American Staffordshire Terrier was referred for the presence of a slow growing cutaneous nodule, located on the right costal area. An FNA was obtained and submitted for analysis. Smears of the aspirate are shown (85a, b; Modified Wright', ×100 oil and ×50 oil, respectively).

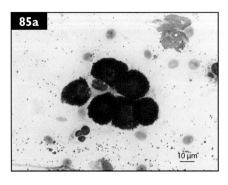
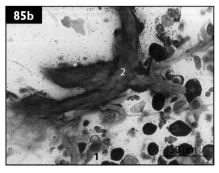

1 Describe the cytologic findings observed in photomicrograph 85a.
2 What is your interpretation?
3 Name the cell labeled 1 and describe the structure labeled 2 in photomicrograph 85b.

CASE 86 An 8-year-old spayed female Akita presented with a chronic cough of 4 months' duration that had not been responsive to antibiotic therapy. The cough was productive and the owner reported that the dog frequently coughed up mucus. Radiographs revealed a combined interstitial, alveolar, and bronchial pattern. A CBC revealed a moderate eosinophilia ($3.4 \times 10^9/l$ [RI = $0.1–1.3 \times 10^9/l$]). A tracheal wash was performed and cytospin preparations made of the material obtained. The microphotograph illustrates a microscopic field representative of the tracheal wash cytology (86; Wright's, ×100).

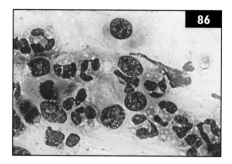

1 What are your differential diagnoses?
2 What other diagnostic test(s) do you recommend?

CASE 87 Uterine cytology was performed for routine assessment when a 7-year-old mare that had her third foal last year arrived at the stud farm prior to breeding (87a, b; both Papanicolaou stain, ×100 oil).

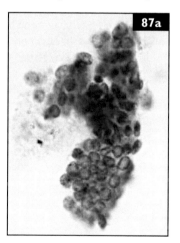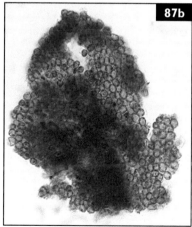

1 Describe what you see in these smears.
2 What is your interpretation of these findings?
3 Why is this good to know?

CASE 88 A 14-year-old neutered male mixed-breed dog, with a history of mild, macrocytic and normochromic, slightly regenerative anemia was presented for investigation of an enlarged and hypoechoic liver. Smears from an aspirate from the liver are shown (88a, b; May–Grünwald–Giemsa, ×40 and ×60, respectively).

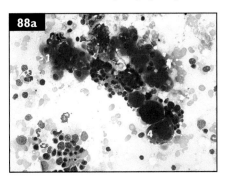
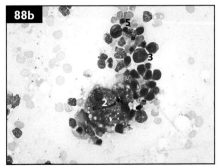

1 Describe the features shown in the photomicrographs, and provide a general description.
2 What is your final interpretation?

CASE 89 A 9-year-old neutered male German Shepherd Dog was presented with a few days history of decreased level of activity, occasional lameness of both hindlimbs, and a stiff gait that worsened after exercise. The dog showed clinical improvement with NSAID treatment. On physical examination there was pain on palpation of both tarsal joints. A synovial fluid specimen was collected and submitted for analysis. Macroscopically the fluid was clear, viscosity was mildly decreased, and mucin clot formation was fair. Fluid analysis revealed: RBCs = 20.0 × 10^9/l; NCC = 52.2 × 10^9/l; TP = 20 g/l. A smear prepared from synovial fluid obtained by fine needle aspiration of the left tarsal joint is shown (89; Modified Wright's, ×50 oil).

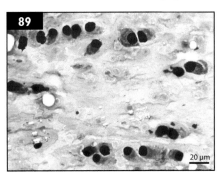

1 What cell types can be identified in the photomicrograph, and how would you describe this cell arrangement?
2 What is your diagnosis?

CASE 90 A 2-year-old DSH cat presented with a history of coughing and gagging that appeared progressive and worsening in intensity. The cat was up-to-date on all vaccinations. A CBC with differential revealed a modest eosinophilia; there were no biochemical abnormalities. Thoracic radiographs revealed a diffuse interstitial pattern with focal peribronchial densities. A transtracheal wash was performed and smears made (**90a, b**; Wright–Giemsa, ×10 and ×50 oil, respectively).

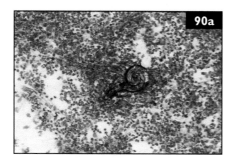 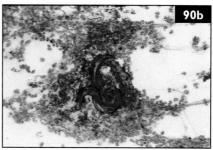

1 What are the main differentials with this pulmonary pattern, cytologic findings, and peripheral eosinophilia?

CASE 91 A 17-year-old Quarter Horse broodmare presented with unilateral mammary gland enlargement. The swollen gland was firm and slightly painful. An FNA was collected from the gland. A smear of the aspirate is shown (**91**; Papanicolaou, ×100 oil).

1 Describe the cells and features seen in the smear.
2 What is your interpretation of this aspirate?

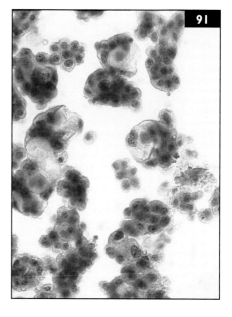

45

CASE 92 A 6-year-old spayed female Shih Tzu was presented with a history of vomiting, weight loss, and depression. Enlarged submandibular and popliteal lymph nodes were detected on physical examination. An FNA from the submandibular node was obtained. Smears of the aspirate are shown (92a, b; May–Grünwald–Giemsa, ×40 and ×100 oil, respectively).

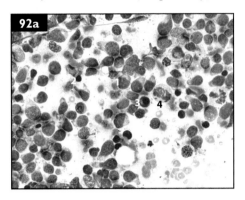 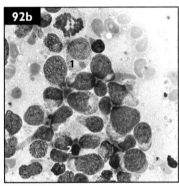

1 Describe the cells represented in the photomicrographs.
2 What is your interpretation?
3 Which is the likely immunophenotype?

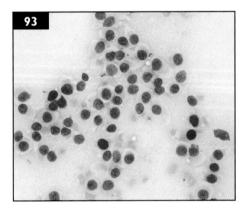

CASE 93 A 1-year-old male West Highland White Terrier was referred for evaluation of a fast growing, ulcerated nodule on the head. The nodule was 1 cm × 1 cm and was located in the parietal area of the head; it was firm, well-circumscribed, and limited to the skin, without adherence to underlying tissues. The dog was otherwise in good health condition. A smear from an aspirate from the head nodule is shown (93; Wright–Giemsa, ×50 oil).

1 Describe the findings seen in the photomicrograph.
2 What is your interpretation? What is the most likely origin of these cells?
3 What would be your therapeutic recommendation in the present case?

CASE 94 An 8-year-old crossbred dog has a history of crusting, flaky skin lesions, weight loss, lethargy, and polyarthropathy. There is generalized, moderate lymphadenopathy. The dog was imported from Spain 18 months previously. Smears from FNAs from two lymph nodes are shown (**94a, b**; both Giemsa, ×100 oil).

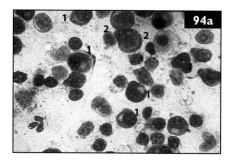 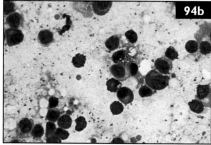

1 What cell(s) are increased in number in **94a**?
2 What does this indicate?
3 What is the cell next to the arrow in **94b**?
4 Given the history and clinical signs, can you speculate on a possible cause for the generalized lymphadenopathy?

CASE 95 A 10-year-old crossbred bitch presented with hematuria that was nonresponsive to antibiotic therapy. A midstream, voided, urine sample was collected for initial analysis. Many epithelial cells were noted on examination of the urinary sediment. A smear of the sediment is shown (**95a**; Wright–Giemsa, ×100 oil).

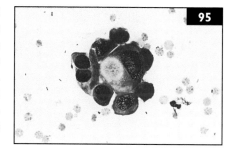

1 Describe the cells identified.
2 What is your provisional diagnosis?
3 What other tests may provide supportive evidence or a definitive diagnosis?
4 What prognosis is associated with this diagnosis?

47

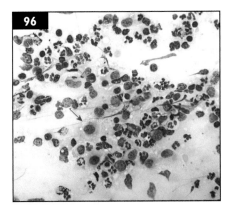

CASE 96 A 3-month-old female Labrador Retriever was presented for an acute onset of facial swelling and bilateral enlargement of submandibular lymph nodes. Fine needle aspiration of submandibular lymph nodes was performed. A smear of the aspirate is shown (**96**; Wright–Giemsa, ×50 oil).

1 Describe the cells shown in the photomicrograph.
2 What are your differential diagnoses based on the history and these cytologic findings?

CASE 97 A 12-year-old male German Bloodhound was presented with a few days history of general signs of illness (fever, lethargy, and emesis), tenesmus, hematuria, and locomotor problems with stiffness of the hindlimbs. On rectal palpation, a slightly painful ventrolateral mass was detected. Ultrasound examination revealed a hypoechoic, encapsulated, fluid-filled lesion within the right lobe of the prostate. The dog received antibiotic therapy for 3 days, 1 week before this sample was taken. Ultrasound-guided fine needle aspiration was performed. A smear of the aspirate is shown (**97**; May–Grünwald–Giemsa, ×100 oil).

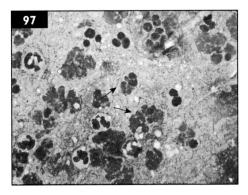

1 Identify the cell population present in the smear, and describe the most relevant characteristics.
2 What is your final interpretation?
3 What additional tests are recommended to confirm the hypothesis?

CASE 98 A 9-year-old entire male dog was presented with a history of a gingival mass. Clinical examination revealed a mass on the buccal aspect of the left mandible above the last molar and an enlarged left mandibular lymph node. Smears from an FNA of the lymph node are shown (**98a, b**; May–Grünwald–Giemsa, ×40 and ×100 oil, respectively).

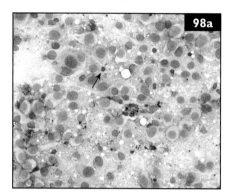
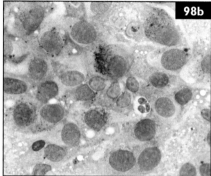

1 Describe the cytologic findings, and give your cytologic interpretation.

CASE 99 A 10-year-old neutered male Rottweiler has a cutaneous mass on the 3rd digit of its left hind foot. The mass has been present for 3 weeks and is growing. The mass is dark red and the skin is hairless. An FNA is collected. A smear of the aspirate is shown (**99**; Giemsa, ×100 oil).

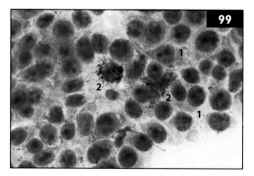

1 Examine the nuclei – are there any criteria of malignancy?
2 Examine the cytoplasm – are there granules present?
3 What is your interpretation?
4 What would you do next?

49

CASE 100 A 2-year-old Labrador Retriever was involved in a road traffic accident. He sustained no fractures and was treated only for shock. Over the following 3 weeks there was a slow but progressive increase in abdominal size and the dog became depressed. Abdominocentesis produced approximately 5 liters of dark green/brown fluid (**100a**). The fluid was submitted to a diagnostic laboratory where a direct smear was made for cytologic examination (**100b**; Wright–Giemsa, ×100 oil).

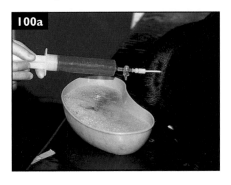

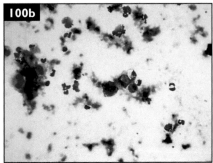

1 Describe the background of the smear.
2 Identify the cells present.
3 What is your provisional diagnosis, and what other tests may be used to confirm this diagnosis?

CASE 101 A 12-year-old neutered male English Setter presented with an oral cavity mass observed by the owner a few days previously. The mass was 3 cm in diameter,

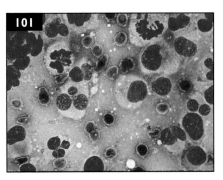

firm and elastic, smooth and pink, and involved the maxilla. A fine needle capillary sampling (puncture without aspiration) was performed. A smear of the sample is shown (**101**; Diff-Quik®, ×100 oil).

1 Identify the cell population present in the smear, and describe the most relevant characteristics.

2 What differential diagnoses would you consider?
3 What additional tests might be recommended?

CASE 102 A 6-year-old spayed female West Highland White Terrier presented with a recent history of seizures and difficulty walking. On clinical examination the dog was ataxic with some postural deficits on all four limbs. MRI revealed hyperintense lesions in the brainstem and parts of the spinal cord. A sample of CSF from the cisterna magna was collected. Both the cell count (125 cells/μl [RI = <5 cells/μl]) and protein concentration (0.6 g/l [RI = <0.3 g/l]) were increased. Smears of the sample are shown (**102a, b**; May–Grünwald–Giemsa, ×10 and ×50 oil, respectively).

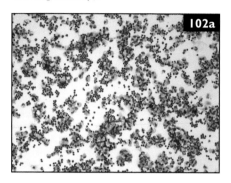
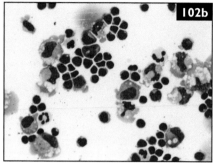

1 What is the cytologic interpretation of this CSF?
2 What are the possible differential diagnoses?

CASE 103 A 10-year-old spayed female barn cat presented with severe dyspnea and cyanosis. Thoracocentesis yielded a foul-smelling, purulent, gray material. A smear of the material is shown (**103**; Gram, ×100 oil).

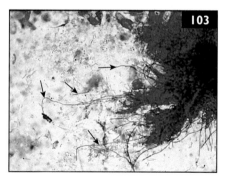

1 What are the structures indicated by the arrows?
2 List two organisms that have this kind of morphology.
3 How can you differentiate between the two before culture results can be received?

51

CASE 104 A 9-year-old female Samoyed presents with dysuria and hematuria. Urinalysis of a free-catch sample reveals pyuria, hematuria, bacteriuria, and numerous, variably sized transitional cells demonstrating multinucleation and anisokaryosis. Palpation and contrast cystography reveal a poorly defined mass in the trigone area of the bladder. A slide is prepared from material obtained following ultrasound-guided fine needle aspiration (**104**; Wright's, ×100 oil).

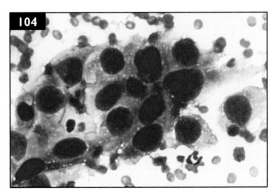

1 What is the most likely diagnosis?

CASE 105 A 6-year-old neutered male Poodle presented with a solitary, firm dermal mass on the shoulder. An FNA of the lesion was obtained. A smear of the aspirate is shown (**105**; Wright–Giemsa, ×20).

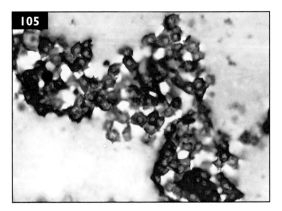

1 What are the structures seen in the smear, and what are they called?
2 What are your main differential diagnoses?

CASE 106 A 7-year-old neutered male Labrador Retriever presented with a history of lethargy and anorexia. Clinical examination was unremarkable. Biochemistry analysis showed: ALT = 97 U/l (RI = 22–78 U/l); total bilirubin = 14.1 μmol/l (RI = 2.4–4.4 μmol/l). Abdominal ultrasound revealed a diffuse increased echogenicity of hepatic parenchyma. An FNA was collected. A smear of the aspirate is shown (**106**; May–Grünwald–Giemsa, ×100 oil).

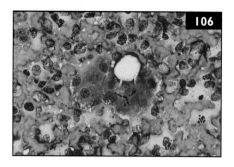

1 Describe the cells seen in the photomicrograph.
2 What is your interpretation?
3 What additional tests might be useful in order to stage the disease?

CASE 107 Identify the exogenous and possible foreign body material in the photomicrograph (**107**; Wright–Giemsa, ×100 oil).

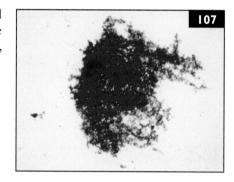

CASE 108 An 8-month-old neutered male Staffordshire Terrier-cross presented with patchy alopecia and erythema on its limbs and head. A skin scrape was made (**108**; 1 = egg; 2 = nymph; 3 = adult; unstained in mineral oil, ×10)

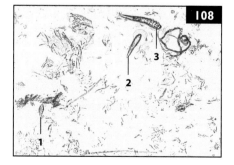

1 What is the organism shown?
2 Why is it important to see multiple life stages?

53

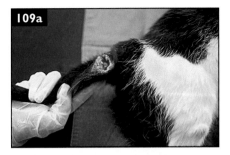

CASE 109 A 5-year-old DSH cat has a number of firm nodular masses up to 3 cm in diameter in the subcutaneous tissue of the back, flanks, and tail. Some are ulcerated (109a). An FNA is collected. Smears of the aspirate are shown (109b, c; Wright–Giemsa, ×50 oil and ×100 oil, respectively).

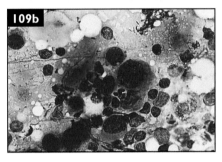

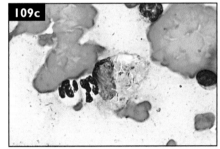

1 What cells are present?
2 What is your interpretation?

CASE 110 A 4-year-old spayed female mixed-breed dog was found locked in a car on a hot summer day. Hematology and biochemistry profiles indicated marked

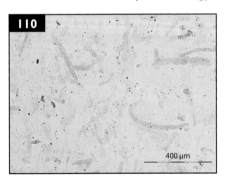

hemoconcentration and azotemia. The dog received parenteral fluids. The next day a urine sample (obtained by cystocentesis) was collected and submitted for analysis. Urine appears pale, yellow, and clear. Analysis revealed: USG = 1.020 (RI = 1.020-1.045); pH = 6.5 (RI = 5.0-7.0). Dipstick evaluation showed traces of protein and bilirubin. A photomicrograph of the urine sediment is shown (110; Wright–Giemsa, ×10)?

1 What are the structures seen on the photomicrograph?
2 How can their visibility be improved?
3 Explain how those structures likely formed in this case.

CASE 111 A 12-year-old cat presented with a subcutaneous, irregular, fluctuating swelling of the right side of the neck and right forelimb. Direct smears of the fluid collected from the lesion were stained for cytologic examination (**111a, b**; Wright–Giemsa, ×40 and ×100 oil, respectively).

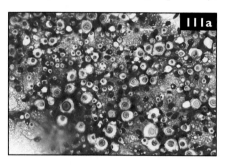
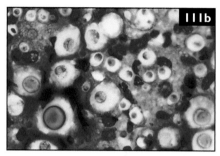

1 Identify the cell populations present, and describe the other features in this field.
2 Classify the inflammatory response present. Does this provide any help with regard to the origin of the structures present in this field?
3 What is your provisional diagnosis, and how might this be confirmed?

CASE 112 A 4-year-old Thoroughbred show jumper is referred for evaluation of a chronic cough and possible decreased performance. A tracheal washing is collected by endoscope and submitted for cytologic evaluation (**112**; Papanicolaou, ×100 oil).

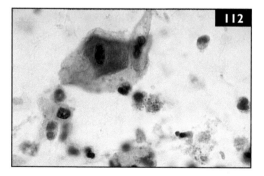

1 What cells and structures can you identify in the photomicrograph?
2 Other fields in the cytologic preparation failed to demonstrate any macrophages or columnar or cuboidal epithelial cells. The features in the photomicrograph are representative of the entire smear. What is your conclusion?

CASE 113 A 9-year-old male German Shepherd Dog presented with a history of intermittent hematuria, dysuria, and tenesmus. At rectal palpation, a nonpainful, symmetrically and slightly enlarged prostate was detected. A prostate FNA was collected. Smears of the aspirate are shown (**113a, b**; May–Grünwald–Giemsa, ×40 and ×100 oil, respectively).

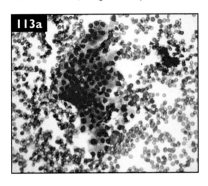 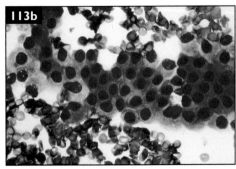

1 Identify the cell population present in the smears, and describe the most relevant characteristics.
2 What is your final interpretation?
3 What are the different methods for collecting cytologic samples from the prostate gland?

CASE 114 An 8-year-old neutered male mixed-breed dog presented with a submandibular swelling. At clinical examination, submandibular and prescapular

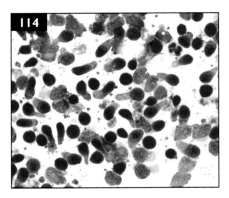

lymph nodes were enlarged and hematology revealed leukocytosis and lymphocytosis. An FNA of the mass was obtained. A smear of the aspirate is shown (**114**; May–Grünwald–Giemsa, ×100 oil).

1 Describe the cells shown in the photomicrograph.
2 What is your interpretation?
3 What further tests would you recommend to reach a definitive diagnosis?

56

CASE 115 A 1-year-old Staffordshire Bull Terrier presented with a hard dry cough that had progressed to hemoptysis. Thoracic radiographs revealed a miliary interstitial pattern. A bronchoalveolar lavage was performed. Smears from the wash are shown (**115a, b**; Wright–Giemsa, ×50 oil and ×100 oil, respectively).

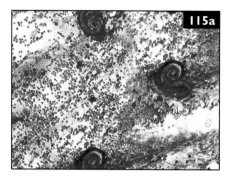
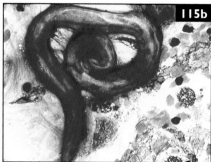

1 How would you describe the wash, and what are the coiled structures in **115a**?
2 At higher magnification these larvae demonstrate kinked tails (**115b**). What are the most likely differentials in dogs? If similar larvae were identified in cats, what is the most likely differential?
3 Is an intermediate host required in the life cycle of *Filaroides* species? If so, name the species, and if not, comment why.
4 How would you confirm the diagnosis?

CASE 116 A 10-year-old Warmblood-cross gelding is referred for evaluation of worsening clinical signs associated with obstructive pulmonary disease/recurrent airway obstruction. A tracheal washing is collected by endoscope and a smear prepared (**116**; Papanicolaou, ×25).

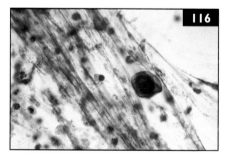

1 What is the structure in the central right portion of the photomicrograph?
2 What is its significance in a respiratory cytology specimen?

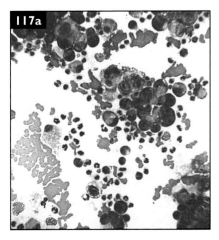

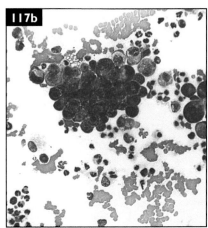

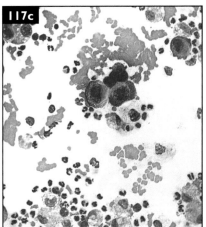

CASE 117 A 9-year-old spayed female Pug presented with a history of coughing, hemoptysis, and dyspnea. A bronchial washing was collected. Smears from the washing are shown (117a–c; all Wright–Giemsa, ×50 oil).

1 Describe the cells shown in the three photomicrographs.
2 What is your interpretation of these findings?
3 What comment would you make about this condition?

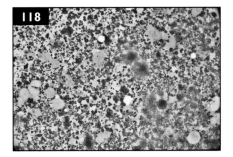

CASE 118 Identify the exogenous and possible foreign body material in this photomicrograph (118; Wright–Giemsa, ×20).

CASE 119 A 6-year-old female Pembroke Welsh Corgi presented with a history of dysorexia and submandibular swelling. At clinical examination, generalized peripheral lymphadenomegaly was noted and an aspirate was collected from the prescapular lymph node. Smears of the aspirate are shown (**119a, b**; May–Grünwald–Giemsa, ×40 and ×100 oil, respectively).

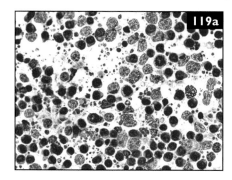 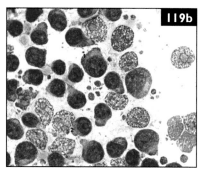

1 Describe the cytologic findings in photomicrograph **119a**.
2 What is your interpretation?
3 What cells are shown in photomicrograph **119b**, and what is the likely immunophenotype?

CASE 120 An 11-year old spayed female Basset Hound presented for evaluation of a 1 cm subcutaneous mass on the right lateral thigh. The mass was soft and freely moveable. A cytology sample from the mass was collected and submitted for analysis. A smear of the sample is shown (**120**; Wright–Giemsa, ×50 oil).

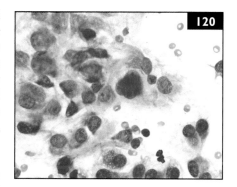

1 The cells in the photomicrograph are most consistent with what general cell lineage?
2 Do these cells exhibit cytologic criteria of malignancy? What is your cytologic interpretation?
3 What is the most likely biological behavior of this type of lesion?

59

CASE 121 A smear from an FNA collected from an 8 cm, partly ulcerated mass on the hindlimb of an 8-year-old Bull Terrier is shown (**121a**; Wright–Giemsa, ×50 oil). The dog was principally presented for melena. The owner had noted the mass previously, but did not think it was important since it occasionally increased in size and then decreased in size. An FNA smear from a different dog with a similar mass is shown (**121b**; Wright–Giemsa, ×100 oil)?

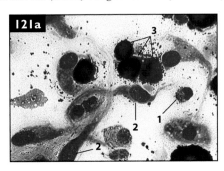
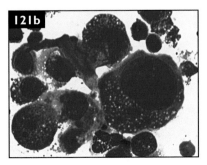

1 Identify the cells labeled 1, 2, and 3 in **121a**. Provide an overall interpretation and explain the significance of these cells within your interpretation.
2 What is the prognosis for the tumor represented in **121a** compared with **121b**?
3 Why is it important to aspirate/biopsy the local lymph node in a confirmed mast cell tumor?

CASE 122 A five-year-old Boxer presented with a history of seizures. Neurologic examination was unremarkable. A cisternal CSF tap was collected. A smear of the CSF is shown (**122**; Wright–Giemsa, ×100 oil).

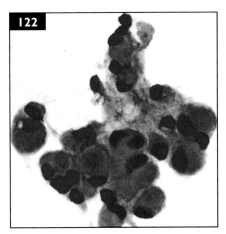

1 What are the cells seen in this photomicrograph, and what is the overall interpretation of this sample?
2 What is their significance in a CSF specimen?

CASE 123 An 8-year-old DLH cat presents with a flat, ulcerated lesion on the upper lip measuring approximately 2 cm × 0.5 cm. Dried blood covers part of the lesion and it is slightly raised. Examination of the mouth reveals an ulcerative lesion on the caudodorsal aspect of the tongue. Fine needle aspiration of the lesion is performed with care. A smear of the aspirate is shown (**123**; Wright's, ×100 oil).

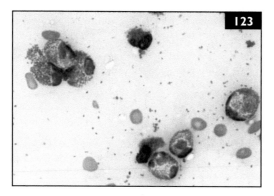

1 What is your interpretation?

CASE 124 A 4-year-old neutered male Corso was presented with a history of anorexia and depression. At clinical examination, mild peripheral lymphadenomegaly and splenomegaly were detected. An FNA was obtained from the prescapular lymph node. A smear of the aspirate is shown (**124**; May–Grünwald–Giemsa, ×100 oil).

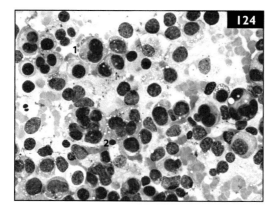

1 Describe the cells shown in the photomicrograph.
2 What is your interpretation?

61

CASE 125 A 9-year-old spayed female Pit Bull with a history of exophthalmos and a swelling over the left eye was referred for a subconjunctival mass extending into the orbit. An aspirate of the mass was submitted for cytologic evaluation. A smear of the aspirate is shown (**125a**; Wright–Giemsa, ×60).

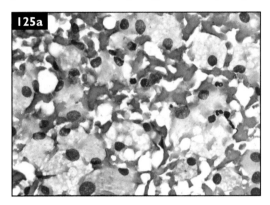

1 Describe the cells shown in the photomicrograph. What is the likely tissue origin of these cells?
2 Is the lesion inflammatory or neoplastic?

CASE 126 A 13-year old spayed female Miniature Poodle presents with two mobile, soft, well-circumscribed, subcutaneous sternal masses, 3 cm and 6 cm in diameter, respectively. The owner had noticed one mass 3 months previously. Fine needle aspiration of both masses is performed and smears are prepared. A representative field of both specimens is illustrated (**126**; Wright's, ×20).

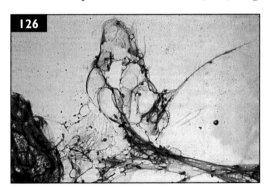

1 What is your interpretation?

CASE 127 A 7-year-old Thoroughbred-cross gelding presented with a history of weight loss. A smear from the sediment from an abdominal fluid specimen is shown (**127**; Wright–Giemsa, ×50 oil).

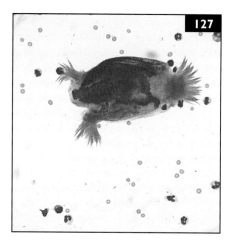

1 What is the structure shown?
2 What is the significance of this finding?
3 What comments do you have regarding this finding?

CASE 128 A 15-year-old spayed female mixed-breed dog was referred to a veterinary practitioner with symptoms of pollakiuria and stranguria. A urine sample was obtained by cystocentesis and submitted for urinalysis and bacterial culture. Urinalysis revealed: USG = 1.022 (RI = 1.020–1.045); pH = 9.0 (RI = 5.0–7.0). Dipstick was strongly positive to blood, moderately positive to leukocytes and nitrite, and showed traces of protein and bilirubin. A smear of the urine sediment is shown (**128**; unstained, ×40).

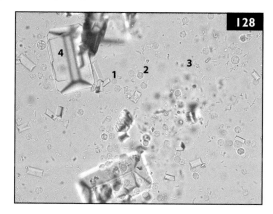

1 Identify the components labeled 1, 2, 3, and 4 in the photomicrograph.
2 What is your interpretation?
3 What is the most likely explanation for the positive reactive of the dipstick to nitrite and the presence of an alkaline pH?

63

CASE 129 A 4-year-old spayed female Alaskan Malamute was presented with a 10-week history of reluctance to stand up and walk, which was intermittent and partially responsive to anti-inflammatory treatment. Physical examination showed severe diffuse joint pain. Radiographs from the carpi did not show signs of erosion or other bone abnormalities. Synovial fluid was obtained by fine needle aspiration from multiple joints (carpi, elbows, and stifles), and all samples showed similar features. The synovial fluid appeared cloudy and had decreased viscosity with poor mucin clot formation. Synovial fluid analysis revealed: TP = 39 g/l (RI = <25 g/l); nucleated cells = 7,300 nucleated cells/μl (RI = <3,000 cells/μl). Samples of synovial fluid were cytocentrifuged and stained (129a, b; both Modified Wright's, ×50 oil).

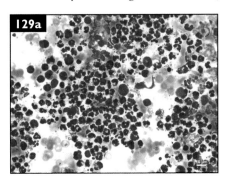

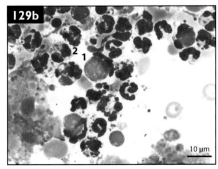

1 Describe the cytologic findings observed in photomicrograph 129a.
2 How would you classify the joint disease?
3 Name the cells labeled 1 and 2 in photomicrograph 129b, and explain their significance.
4 What would be your main differential diagnosis?

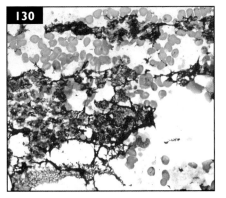

CASE 130 Ultrasound-guided liver aspiration was performed on a 10-year-old neutered male dog with a history of hepatomegaly and high liver enzymes. A smear of the aspirate obtained is shown (130; Modified Wright's, ×50 oil).

1 What is the magenta substance visible in the background of the smear?

CASE 131 A 3-year-old gelding was box walking, sweating, stamping, and head pressing. A sample of peritoneal fluid was collected and examined immediately. It was turbid and serosanguineous and had an NCC of $21 \times 10^9/l$ and a TP of 43 g/l. Cells seen in a cytospin preparation of the fluid are shown (**131**; Wright–Giemsa, ×100 oil).

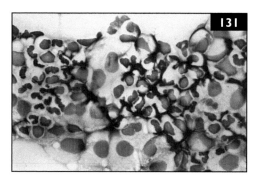

1 What type of fluid is present (fluid classification)?
2 What cells are present?
3 What is your interpretation?

CASE 132 An FNA is collected from a mass on the left shoulder of a 10-year-old female neutered DSH cat. A smear of the aspirate is shown (**132**; Wright–Giemsa ×50 oil).

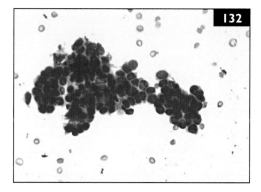

1 Describe the cells shown in the smear.
2 What is your interpretation of these findings?
3 What prognosis do you expect?

65

CASE 133 A 9-year-old neutered male DSH cat presented for evaluation of a 3 cm subcutaneous mass on the left flank. Other medical history included a history of chronic recurrent herpes viral infection, manifested by opacity and neovascularization of the left cornea, intermittent sneezing, and upper respiratory wheezing. Aspirates from the mass were taken and submitted. Smears of the aspirate are shown (**133a, b**; both Wright–Giemsa, ×20).

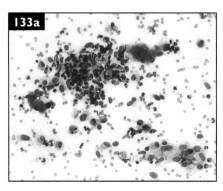 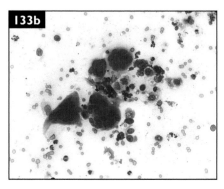

1 Based on the cells present in photomicrograph **133a**, what is the most likely cytologic diagnosis?
2 What are the four extremely large cells seen in photomicrograph **133b**? How should these be interpreted?
3 What etiology should be considered for the mass?

CASE 134 An FNA was collected from a neck mass in a cat. Smears were made and sent to an external veterinary diagnostic laboratory for cytologic examination (**134**; Wright Giemsa, ×50 oil), together with a few other cytologic and histologic samples from different animals.

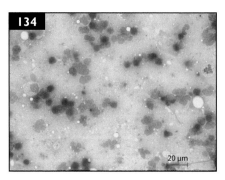

1 What has caused the turquoise–blue, hazy appearance of the slide, and how can this be prevented?

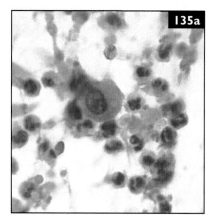

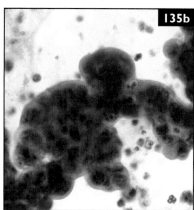

CASE 135 A 19-year-old Clydesdale-cross gelding presented with a history of weight loss, partial anorexia, and mild recurrent colic. An abdominal fluid sample was collected and analysis revealed: NCC = 15 × 10^9/l; TP = 40 g/l. Smears of the fluid are shown (**135a–c; a, b,** Papanicolaou, ×50 oil and ×100 oil, respectively; **109c,** Wright–Giemsa, ×50 oil).

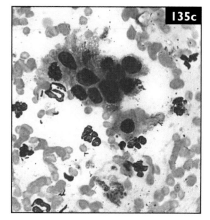

1 Describe the features seen in the photomicrographs.
2 What is your interpretation of this specimen?
3 What is the prognosis for this condition?

CASE 136 A 15-year-old horse was referred for evaluation of a small cutaneous skin lesion in the neck area. An FNA of the mass was obtained. A smear of the aspirate is shown (**136;** Wright–Giemsa, ×50 oil).

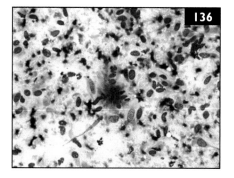

1 Describe the cells shown in the photomicrograph.
2 What are your differential diagnoses based on these cytologic findings?

CASE 137 Bronchoalveolar lavage is performed on a 2-year-old Thoroughbred gelding in racing training presented because of a history of poor performance. A smear of the sediment from the lavage is shown (**137**; Wright–Giemsa, ×100 oil).

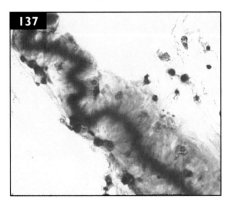

1 What is the structure shown?
2 What is the significance of this finding in a respiratory cytology specimen?

CASE 138 A 14-year-old entire female Yorkshire Terrier presented with a recent history of polyuria/polydipsia and labored breathing. Clinical examination and diagnostic imaging showed mitral valve insufficiency, pulmonary edema, and a 3 cm mass in the left adrenal gland, with caudal vena cava invasion. A smear from an ultrasound-guided aspirate of the mass is shown (**138**; May–Grünwald–Giemsa, ×40).

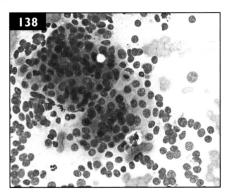

1 Identify the cell population present in the photomicrograph, and describe the most relevant cytologic findings.
2 What is your interpretation of these findings?
3 What additional tests could be used to support and confirm the diagnosis?

CASE 139 A 10-year-old mare arrives at a breeding farm in January without a foal at her side. No previous history is available. A uterine washing is collected to determine the mare's reproductive status. A smear of the washing is shown (**139**; Papanicolaou, ×100 oil).

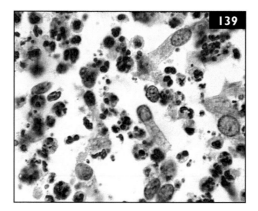

1 Describe the features shown in the smear.
2 What is your interpretation of these findings?

CASE 140 A 3-year-old maiden mare arrives at a breeding farm in May. A uterine washing is collected to assess her reproductive status. A smear of the washing is shown (**140**; Papanicolaou, ×50 oil).

1 Describe the features seen.
2 What is your interpretation of these findings?
3 Why is this important?

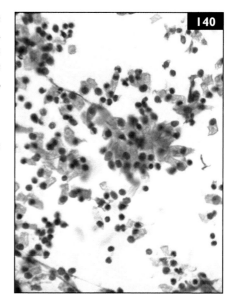

CASE 141 A 7-year-old neutered male Ariège Pointing was presented with a history of a rectal mass. This appeared as a firm, irregular, 3 cm diameter lesion associated with the anal sac. Smears from an FNA of the mass are shown (**141a, b**; May–Grünwald–Giemsa, ×20 and ×100 oil, respectively).

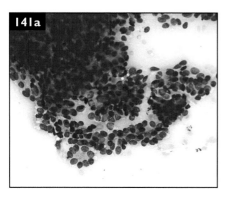
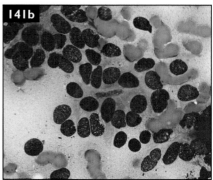

1 Describe the cytologic findings, and give your cytologic interpretation.
2 What additional tests would you recommend?

CASE 142 An 8-year-old entire male Border Terrier presented with a history of blood in the urine. An enlarged, irregularly-shaped prostate gland was felt on palpation. A prostatic washing was collected. A smear of the washing is shown (**142**; Wright–Giemsa, ×100 oil).

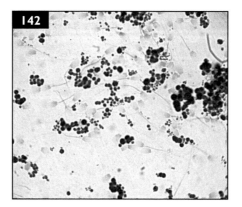

1 Describe the findings in the smear.
2 What is the significance of these findings?
3 What other recommendations might you have?

CASE 143 A 2-year-old neutered male Basset Hound presented with a 3-day history of inappetence; the owners also reported that the dog seemed to yelp when they touched his neck. On clinical examination the dog was pyrexic and had pain on manipulation of the neck. A sample of CSF was collected from the cisterna magna and submitted for analysis. Both cell count (80 cells/µl [RI = <5 cells/µl]) and protein concentration (1.2 g/l [RI = <0.3 g/l]) were increased. Smears of the CSF are shown (**143a, b**; May–Grünwald–Giemsa, ×10 and ×50 oil, respectively).

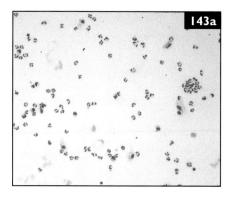
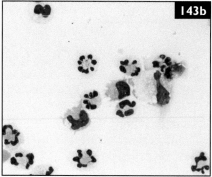

1 What is the cytologic interpretation of this CSF?
2 What are the possible differential diagnoses?

CASE 144 A 5-year-old Thoroughbred-cross gelding presented for a tracheal washing. No history was included regarding the reason for obtaining the wash. A smear of the wash is shown (**144**; Papanicolaou, ×100 oil).

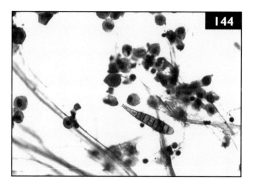

1 What is the elongated, brown, segmented structure in the lower right/central portion of the smear?
2 What is the significance of this finding?

71

CASE 145 A 9-year-old neutered male Cocker Spaniel presented for investigation of a small alopecic mass on the neck. The lesion had been present for several months without change in size. Smears of the mass are shown (**145a, b;** Wright–Giemsa, ×50 oil and ×100 oil, respectively).

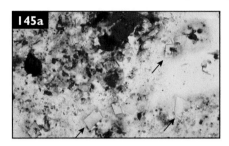 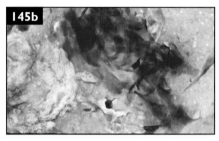

1 Describe the cytologic findings seen in the photomicrographs, and give your interpretation.
2 What are the structures pointed to by the arrows in **145a**. What is the significance of these structures?

CASE 146 A 14-year-old neutered male cat presented for a routine check-up. Hematology was unremarkable; abnormal biochemistry values included: TP = 82 g/l (RI = 61–80 g/l); albumin = 38 g/l (RI = 22–36 g/l). A voided urine sample was brought by the owner directly to the laboratory and submitted for analysis. The urine was dark yellow and turbid. Urinalysis revealed: USG = 1.050 (RI = 1.020–1.060); pH = 8.0 (RI = 5.0–7.0). Urine dipstick was strongly positive for leukocytes and negative for protein. A smear of the urine sediment is shown (**146;** unstained, ×20).

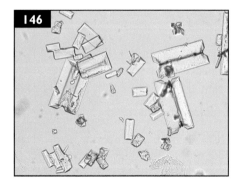

1 What kind of crystals are shown on the photomicrograph?
2 What do they tell you from a clinical point of view with regard to the other findings?

CASE 147 Pleural fluid is obtained from an 8-year-old cat with recent development of dyspnea and pleural effusion (147a). Analysis of the fluid revealed: TP = 52.2 g/l; albumin = 27.5 g/l; globulin = 24.7 g/l; albumin:globulin ratio = 1:1; SG = 1.040; NCC = 54.96 × 10⁹/l; RBCs = 0.28 × 10¹²/l. Smears of the fluid are shown (147b, c; Wright–Giemsa, ×50 oil and ×100 oil, respectively)

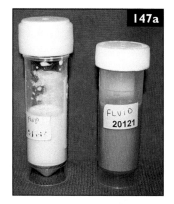
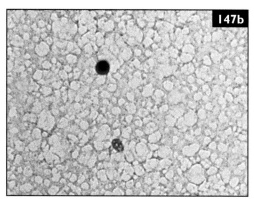

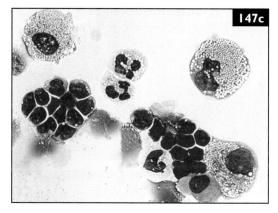

1 Classify the pleural fluid.
2 Based on the macroscopic (147a) and microscopic (147b, c) appearance of the pleural fluid, what further laboratory tests would you like to request?
3 Given the results of the tests requested above, how would you now reclassify this fluid?
4 List the most common causes of chylous effusions in cats.

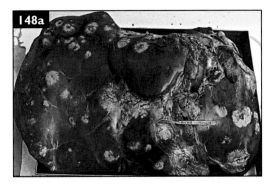

CASE 148 A thin, inappetent 5-year-old Friesian cow was euthanized. On postmortem examination the liver was found to be studded with yellow masses (148a). An impression smear from one of the masses is shown (148b; Wright–Giemsa, ×50 oil).

1 What cells are present?
2 What is the cytologic interpretation?

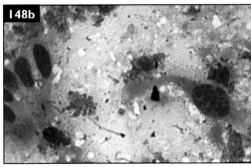

CASE 149 A 3-year-old entire female Shetland Sheepdog presented for depression and apparent blindness. Ophthalmic examination revealed multifocal white–gray discoloration of the retina with increased ocular pressure. A vitreal aspirate was submitted for analysis (149; Wright–Giemsa, ×100 oil).

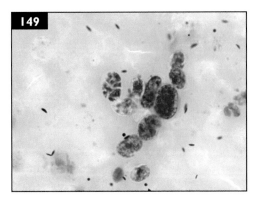

1 Identify the organism.

74

CASE 150 An aspirate is collected from a rapidly growing mass on the left thorax of a 6-year-old entire female Boston Terrier. Smears of the aspirate are shown (**150a, b**; Wright–Giemsa, ×50 oil and ×100 oil, respectively).

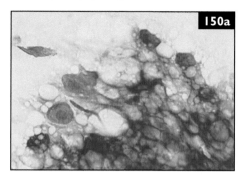
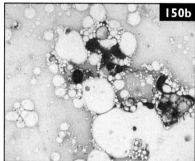

1 Describe the features seen in the smears.
2 What is your cytologic interpretation?
3 Are there any confirmatory tests that can/should be done?

CASE 151 An 11-year-old neutered male DSH cat presented with a history of lethargy and anorexia. Clinical examination revealed icteric mucous membranes. As part of the diagnostic investigation process, a liver aspirate was collected. A smear of the aspirate is shown (**151**; May–Grünwald–Giemsa, ×100 oil).

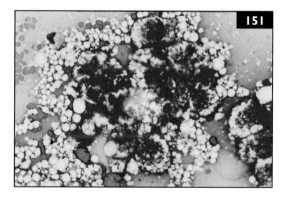

1 Describe the cytologic findings, and give your cytologic interpretation.
2 What are the most frequent causes of this condition?

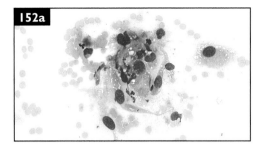

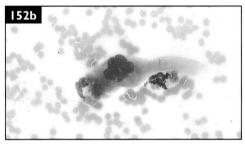

CASE 152 A 6-year-old spayed female Labrador Retriever was initially seen for a soft tissue sarcoma on the forelimb. The mass was incompletely excised. Following surgery, the dog received a radiotherapy cycle. On routine recheck, a small tissue thickening in the area of the surgical scar was noted and an FNA was obtained. Smears of the aspirate are shown (**152a, b**; both Wright–Giemsa, ×100 oil).

1 Describe the cells shown in the images.
2 What is your interpretation and recommendation?

CASE 153 A 5-year-old entire female German Shepherd Dog-cross presents with a history of a chronic mucopurulent nasal discharge for 6 months. A smear from a nasal washing is shown (**153**; Wright–Giemsa, ×100 oil).

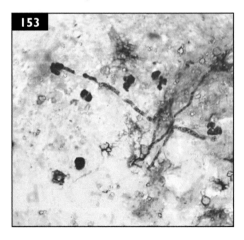

1 Describe the features shown.
2 What is your interpretation of these findings?
3 What additional tests might be recommended?

CASE 154 A 7-year-old spayed female Cocker Spaniel presented with a small alopecic mass on the head. Smears from an aspirate from the mass are shown (**154a, b**; both Wright–Giemsa, ×50 oil).

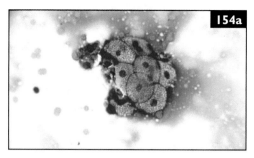

1 What cells are represented in **154a**?
2 What is your diagnosis?
3 What are the cells indicated by the arrows in **154b**. What is the significance of these cells?

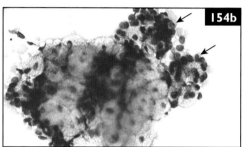

CASE 155 A 6-year-old entire female Jack Russell Terrier was presented with a history of anorexia. Radiographs revealed a thoracic mass occupying the cranial two-thirds of the thoracic cavity, which did not appear to involve the heart or lungs. FNAs of the mass were obtained. A smear of one of the aspirates is shown (**155**; Modified Wright's, ×50 oil)

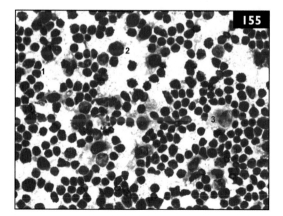

1 What cell types are present in the photomicrograph?
2 What is your interpretation?

CASE 156 A 4-year-old neutered male German Shepherd Dog presented with a history of pyrexia of unknown origin. Clinical examination was unremarkable. A sample of CSF from the cisterna magna was collected. CSF analysis revealed: NCC = 100 cells/µl (RI = <5 cells/µl); CSF protein = 1.14 g/l (RI = <0.3 g/l). Smears of the CSF are shown (**156a, b**; Wright's Giemsa, ×10 and ×50 oil, respectively).

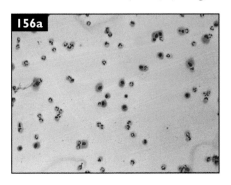
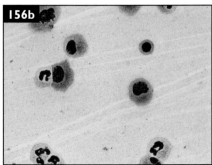

1 What is the cytologic interpretation of this CSF?
2 What are the possible differential diagnoses?

CASE 157 A splenic aspirate was collected from the spleen of a 3-year-old spayed female Dachshund with immune-mediated hemolytic anemia. A smear of the aspirate is shown (**157**; Modified Wright's, ×50 oil).

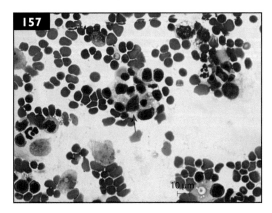

1 What cells are present in the center of the photomicrograph (arrow)?
2 What process does this represent, and when does it occur?

CASE 158 A 3-year-old spayed female crossbred dog presented with a history of a cystic mass in the caudal abdomen. On ultrasonography, the mass did not appear to be associated with any organs. An FNA was obtained. Smears of the aspirate are shown (**158a, b**; Wright–Giemsa, ×20 and ×50 oil, respectively).

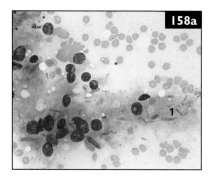 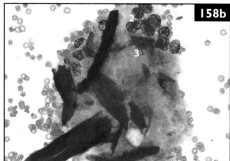

1 Describe the findings seen in the photomicrographs.
2 What is your interpretation?

CASE 159 An FNA is collected from a prescapular lymph node of a 6-year-old Terrier. A smear of the aspirate is shown (**159**; Wright–Giemsa, ×50 oil).

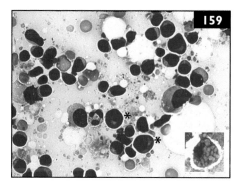

1 Which interpretation best describes this smear:
  (a) normal;
  (b) reactive/hyperplastic;
  (c) metastatic tumor; or
  (d) multiple myeloma?
2 What are Mott cells (see inset) and tingible body macrophages?
3 List the differentials for reactive/hyperplastic lymph nodes.

CASE 160 A 9-year-old neutered male Welsh Pembroke Corgi presented for an 8 cm × 6 cm firm, subcutaneous mass in the dorsal lumbar region adjacent to the left hip. A cytology sample was collected and submitted for analysis. Smears of the sample are shown (**160a, b**; Wright–Giemsa, ×20 and ×50 oil, respectively).

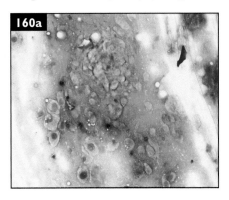
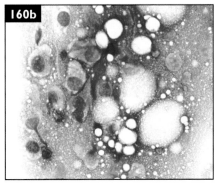

1 Describe the cells and the background material present in the photomicrographs.
2 What is the most likely cytologic diagnosis?

CASE 161 A 7-year-old Cocker Spaniel was presented for restaging of anal sac carcinoma removed 6 months before. Abdominal ultrasound revealed a small hypoechoic hepatic lesion. An FNA was collected and submitted for analysis. A smear of the aspirate is shown (**161**; Wright–Giemsa, ×50 oil).

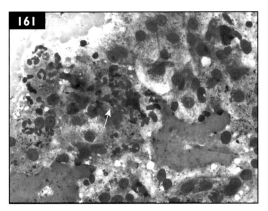

1 Describe the findings seen in the photomicrograph.
2 What is your interpretation based on these cytologic findings?

CASE 162 A 10-year-old entire male German Shepherd Dog was presented for an enlarged right testicle. Fine needle biopsy of the testicle was performed. Smears of the biopsy sample obtained are shown (**162a, b**; May–Grünwald–Giemsa, ×40 and ×60, respectively).

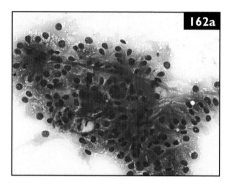 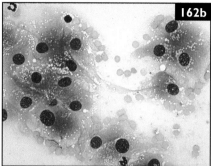

1 Describe the features observed in the photomicrographs, and provide a general description.
2 What is your interpretation?

CASE 163 A 6-year-old spayed female dog was referred for investigation of an enlarged and hyperechoic spleen. Abdominal ultrasound revealed mild splenomegaly. An FNA was collected and submitted for analysis (**163**; Wright–Giemsa, ×100 oil).

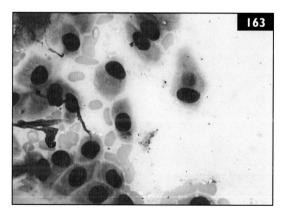

1 What is the likely origin of these cells?

CASE 164 A 6-year-old spayed female Boxer presented with a large mass located in the mammary gland region. The mass measured 4 cm × 3 cm in diameter. It was firm, adherent, and warm. An FNA was obtained. A smear of the aspirate is shown (**164**; Modified Wright's, ×50 oil).

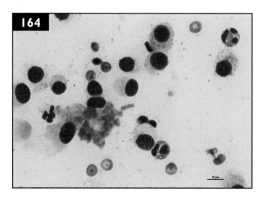

1 Describe the cytologic findings observed in the photomicrograph.
2 What is your interpretation?

CASE 165 An FNA from an irregular, erythematous, cutaneous thickening or mass-like lesion in a dog was collected and submitted for analysis. A smear of the aspirate is shown (**165**; Wright–Giemsa, ×100 oil).

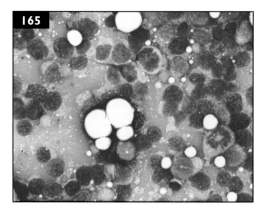

1 Describe the features shown in the photomicrograph.
2 What is your interpretation of these findings?

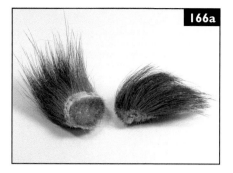

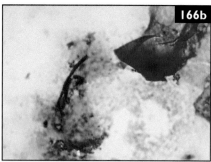

CASE 166 A yearling female Icelandic horse was kept outdoors in a paddock during the winter months and developed skin lesions on the dorsal trunk and flanks. The lesions consisted of raised scabs, 1 cm in diameter, with matted hair. The underside was concave with protruding hair roots. Removal of the lesions was painful for the horse, revealing an exudative dermatitis beneath. Two of the scabs were submitted for examination (**166a**). The material was chopped with a scalpel and macerated in saline. A number of

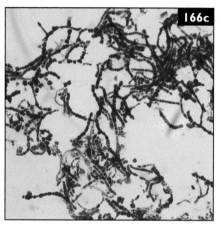

imprints and squash preparations were made and stained with a routine cytology stain as well as Gram stain (**166b, c**; both ×100 oil).

1 What are the organisms shown in the photomicrographs?
2 How are they identified?
3 What are the differentials?

83

CASE 1

1 Identify the cell population present in the smear. The samples are of good cellularity and contain a main population of discrete cells, arranged in poorly cohesive groups. These cells have a histiocytoid appearance, with abundant pale blue cytoplasm and poorly distinct borders. Nuclei are round to oval, eccentrically located, and contain reticular chromatin and one or two prominent, round nucleoli. Scattered eosinophils are noted among these cells. Several free orange granules are also seen in the background.

2 What is your interpretation? The round cell population observed is suggestive of either histiocytes or poorly granulated mast cells. Additional histochemical and immunohistochemical staining is recommended to investigate this further; this may include Toluidine Blue and CD117 and will help to confirm/exclude a possible mast cell origin. In this case, the signalment and the cytologic appearance of these cells are primarily suggestive of a histiocytic variant of a feline mast cell tumor (MCT). This rare sub-type of MCT has been described mainly in young Siamese cats and commonly presents as multiple cutaneous/subcutaneous nodules on the trunk, head, and limbs. Cytologically, poorly granulated mast cells with a histiocytic appearance are the main cellular population; eosinophils can also be observed. The prognosis for this form of MCT is usually good, since spontaneous regression frequently occurs. Six months from the onset of the first lesions, this cat recovered and all the lesions disappeared without any treatment.

Further reading
Wilcock BP, Yager JA, Zink MC (1986) The morphology and behavior of feline cutaneous mastocytomas. *Veterinary Pathology* **23**:320–324.

CASE 2

1 Describe the cells seen. There are scattered erythrocytes and many individual cells with oval nuclei, coarse granular chromatin, often containing one to several prominent round nucleoli. The cytoplasm is moderate in amounts, basophilic, frequently elongated, forming cytoplasmic tails. There are several very large multinucleated cells whose nuclei have the same features as the mononucleated cells.

2 What is your cytologic interpretation? Mesenchymal proliferation, primarily suggestive of a soft tissue sarcoma.

3 What differential diagnoses would you consider? Differential diagnoses that should be considered are:
- Severe reactive fibroplasia: unlikely given the history of a distinct mass, the absence of inflammatory cells, and the presence of significant cytologic features of atypia.

- Soft tissue sarcoma: histopathology is required for further characterization. Possible differentials include: (a) fibrosarcoma; (b) anaplastic sarcoma with giant cells (given the presence of multinucleated elements).

In this case, there was subsequent identification of radiographic evidence of bone involvement. When removed, the tumor could be seen to be arising from the periosteum and small islands of osteoid were also seen. Therefore, the histologic diagnosis was giant cell sarcoma of bone.

CASE 3

1 What process is observed in the photomicrograph? Leukocytophagia, which is the phagocytosis of leukocytes (in this specific case neutrophils) by macrophages. The latter appear reactive and are characterized by abundant foamy cytoplasm, with poorly defined clear vacuoles. Leukocytophagia is a nonspecific process frequently observed in association with chronic inflammation.

CASE 4

1 How would you classify this fluid? Modified transudate.

2 What cell types can be seen in the photomicrograph? A few erythrocytes and high numbers of neutrophils. In the center of the field there are two cells with features of malignancy. One is small and mononucleated and the other is large and contains multiple nuclei, several of which are not in the plane of focus. The nuclei often contain uneven nuclear membrane thickening and distinct nucleoli. The cytoplasm has a crisply defined border and central dense character, with a more delicate periphery of endoplasmic and ectoplasmic differentiation, which is consistent with squamous differentiation.

3 What is your interpretation? Squamous cell carcinoma (SCC) of the stomach. The neutrophilic response is characteristic for this type of tumor. Squamous epithelial cells are found in peritoneal fluid when the tumor has caused rupture or ulceration of the stomach wall and communication with the peritoneal cavity, or when there has been lymphatic metastasis, often with ulceration or rupture of lymphatics that allow cells into the peritoneal cavity. Therefore, neoplastic cells may not be apparent in all cases with gastric SCC and their detection will depend on the stage of the disease, its progression, and the number of cells shed into the peritoneal cavity. Neoplastic cells may fail to be represented in smears or may be missed or masked by inflammation or hemorrhage if present only in small numbers.

SCC of the stomach in the horse has a poor prognosis since it is often not diagnosed until advanced disease and/or metastasis is present. Endoscopic evaluation is often helpful in the diagnosis of esophageal or gastric SCC, particularly if neoplastic cells are not apparent in the peritoneal fluid. Washings of the stomach or brushings of suspicious lesions have also been used successfully in the diagnosis of gastric SCC in the horse when peritoneal fluid was not rewarding in demonstrating neoplastic cells.

Further reading
Cowell RL, Tyler RD (2002) (eds) *Diagnostic Cytology and Hematology of the Horse*, 2nd edn. Mosby, St. Louis.

CASE 5

1 Classify the fluid based on the photomicrographs and the laboratory data. Modified transudate, a category combining both properties of transudates (NCC $<1 \times 10^9$/l) and exudates (TP >30g/l). At low magnification, the background is finely granular with lighter staining crescent artifacts. This background suggests increased globular protein concentration (**5b**).

2 Interpret the electrophoresis trace. Electrophoresis reveals: (1) alpha-2 spike consistent with an acute phase response: proteins in the alpha-2 region are produced by the liver in response to a network of cytokines involved in inflammation; and (2) a marked polyclonal elevation of gamma globulins consistent with a polyclonal gammopathy. Overall, electrophoresis is consistent with a marked, established inflammatory process.

3 Although the electrophoresis pattern is not pathognomonic for specific conditions, in the context of the other findings in this particular case, what diagnosis should be at the top of the differential list? Feline infectious peritonitis (FIP). A tentative clinical diagnosis of FIP is based on multiple strong positive results in a panel of tests: appropriate clinical signs (e.g. ascites, age [young]); fluid albumin:globulin ratio <0.8; high fluid and plasma globulin concentrations; electrophoresis (trace in this case is classic); positive coronavirus antibody on fluid or serum/plasma (this patient was FIP/coronavirus positive with a titer of 1:2,560 [ELISA test]).

Editors' note: A well-known adage regarding FIP is that it is a 'diagnosis of exclusion and support' when suggestive cytologic findings are present. Other possible causes of effusion need to be excluded, while additional supporting evidence for FIP is needed. FIP is typically a disease of young (<2 years of age) or older cats. Hypergammaglobulinemia is frequently present, as well as albumin:globulin ratios of <0.8 in serum and effusion fluids. Polyclonal gammopathies with similar protein electrophoresis findings in serum and peritoneal fluid are supportive. Lymphopenia is often present. A positive titer for feline coronavirus does not provide support for this diagnosis since many cats without disease will have positive titers. The level of antibody titer is not of diagnostic or prognostic significance. A negative titer in a healthy cat suggests that the cat has not been exposed to feline coronavirus. A negative titer in a sick cat does not rule out FIP since some cats with fulminant FIP may present with negative titers due to anergy or antigen–antibody complex formation that limits the ability to detect antibodies to this virus.

Further reading

Pedersen NC (1995) An overview of feline enteric coronavirus and feline infectious peritonitis. *Feline Practice* 23(3):7.

Pedersen NC (2014) An update on feline infectious peritonitis: diagnostics and therapeutics. *Veterinary Journal* 201(2):133–141.

Sparkes AH, Gruffydd-Jones TJ, Harbour DA (1994) An appraisal of the value of laboratory tests in the diagnosis of feline infectious peritonitis. *Journal of the American Animal Hospital Association* 30:345–350.

CASE 6

1 Describe the cells shown in the photomicrograph. The photomicrograph shows an increased number of pleomorphic, large roundish cells with moderate amounts of lightly granular basophilic cytoplasm and well-defined cytoplasmic borders. Nuclei are round, central to paracentral, large, with granular chromatin and poorly distinct nucleoli. A few binucleated and trinucleated cells (not seen in this photomicrograph) were also noted. Anisocytosis and anisokaryosis are moderate with one atypical mitotic figure seen. The cytologic interpretation is malignant neoplasia of unknown origin. The main differentials are primary or metastatic tumor of the CNS, histiocytic neoplasia, and lymphoma.

2 What are your differential diagnoses based on these cytologic findings, and what additional tests would you recommend? Additional investigations are

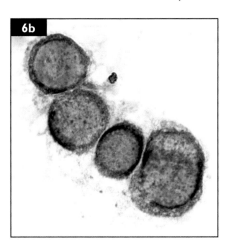

6b

recommended in this case to further characterize the lesion, and may include histopathology (not possible in this case given the location of the lesion) and immunostaining. Immunocytochemistry (6b; cytokeratin, ×100 oil) shows strong positivity to cytokeratin and is negative for vimentin, CD3, CD79a, and CD18. These findings are consistent with carcinoma, probably metastatic mammary carcinoma, given the history of previous mammary carcinoma.

Cells from metastatic carcinoma with a discrete round cell appearance have been reported in CSF samples from humans and dogs; the reason for this remains unclear, but downregulation of adhesion molecules on the cell membranes of neoplastic cells is a possibility.

Editors' note: Given this lack of clustering of epithelial cells in CSF, immunostaining is considered to be a useful diagnostic tool for the identification of the cellular lineage in CSF samples.

Further reading
Behling-Kelly E, Petersen S, Muthuswamy A *et al.* (2010) Neoplastic pleocytosis in a dog with metastatic mammary carcinoma and meningeal carcinomatosis. *Veterinary Clinical Pathology* **39**:247–252.

CASE 7

1 What cells are present? There is a mixed population of nucleated cells, including neutrophils, macrophages, and lymphocytes. There are also intracytoplasmic rod-shaped bacteria.
2 What is your interpretation? The cytologic interpretation is mixed, mostly neutrophilic septic inflammation; bacterial culture confirmed growth of *Actinobacillus* species.

CASE 8

1 Describe the organisms seen. There is a mixed population of gram-negative rods, gram-positive rods and small cocci, and gram-positive rounded rods with central spores that often distend the sporangium (the middle of the bacteria).
2 Are the spore-forming gram-positive rods likely to be *Clostridium perfringens*? No. *C. perfringens* are gram-positive spore-forming rods, but they are classically square-ended and the central spore does not distend the sporangium. These are more likely to be *Bacillus* species, a huge group of aerobic gram-positive spore formers that are common in the environment. Many have rapid generation times and can overgrow in diarrheic stool; they may be able to thrive where other organisms are purged by the rapid transit. The similarities between these two genera, cytologically, may contribute to the controversy regarding the role of *C. perfringens* in diarrhea.

Editors' note: Whenever gram-positive, spore-forming rods are seen in a fecal smear and *C. perfringens* or *Bacillus* species is suspected, confirmation by culture and/or endotoxin assay should be considered in order to provide a definitive diagnosis.

Answers

CASE 9

1 Describe the findings seen in the photomicrograph. The aspirate harvested a monomorphic population of round cells in a clear to mildly granular background, with rare RBCs. The round cells have moderate amounts of blue cytoplasm, occasionally showing a clear perinuclear halo, and discrete cytoplasmic borders. Nuclei are round, eccentrically located, with coarsely clumped chromatin pattern, and some nuclei can be seen to contain small round nucleoli. Anisocytosis and anisokaryosis are moderate; rare binucleated cells are seen.

2 What is your interpretation? Plasmacytoma. This is a benign plasma cell tumor of the skin observed in dogs and, only rarely, in cats. Treatment involves wide surgical excision. Prognosis is generally good, although recurrence may be observed. In poorly differentiated forms, cytology may not be sufficient to reach a definitive diagnosis and additional investigations may be required. Plasma cells express markers typical of B lymphoid cells, including CD79a, lambda chain, and MUM1 (the latter specific for plasma cells). All these can be tested with several diagnostic techniques including immunocytochemistry, immunohistochemistry, and flow cytometry.

Editors' note: In poorly differentiated plasmacytomas, it may be impossible to differentiate a cutaneous plasmacytoma from either a cutaneous histiocytoma or a lymphoma. Cutaneous plasmacytomas and lymphomas tend to occur in middle aged to older dogs, while histiocytomas can occur in any age group, but are particularly common in young dogs. Histopathology and immunochemical methods, as indicated above, are useful in differentiating these tumors.

CASE 10

1 What features are shown? High numbers of erythrocytes, a large clump of platelets (center), and a few leukocytes.

2 What is the significance of these findings in an abdominal effusion? The findings are consistent with the presence of fresh blood. Usually, platelets disappear from fresh hemorrhage within 2–4 hours. Their presence supports very recent hemorrhage and/or contamination with blood during the procedure.

CASE 11

1 What is the most likely origin of the cell population? The predominant population consists of medium to large sized, ovoid-shaped cells, with distinct cytoplasmic borders arranged in clusters and sheets, overall suggestive of an epithelial origin.

2 Which criteria of malignancy do these cells demonstrate? These cells show multiple criteria of malignancy, including marked anisocytosis and anisokaryosis, multinucleation, multiple prominent nucleoli, and increased N:C ratio. Some cells also have a 'signet ring' appearance. The latter is a cytologic feature commonly observed in some types of carcinomas and characterized by the presence of a large intracytoplasmic vacuole that pushes the nucleus to the side of the cell periphery, giving to the cell this characteristic shape.

3 What is your interpretation of these findings? The cytologic features of this aspirate are compatible with a malignant epithelial neoplasia (carcinoma). A dysplastic/neoplastic proliferation of mesothelial cells is another possible differential diagnosis (e.g. reactive mesothelium, mesothelioma). Postmortem examination confirmed the presence of a pancreatic adenocarcinoma with metastases to the mesentery and liver.

Editors' note: In effusion samples, the distinction between neoplastic epithelial cells (carcinomatosis) and dysplastic/neoplastic mesothelial cells is frequently not possible. The presence of tight junctions within cell groups is supportive of epithelial origin, while 'windows' or slits between cells within groups are more supportive of a mesothelial origin. Additional elements that may help in the diagnostic process include a detailed clinical history/examination (presence of a primary mass, which may lean towards a diagnosis of carcinoma), together with histopathologic and/or immunohistochemical findings (carcinomas tend to be cytokeratin positive and vimentin negative, whereas mesotheliomas frequently co-express both markers).

CASE 12

1 What cells are present? There is a pleomorphic population of squamous epithelial cells. These vary from elongated forms with indefinite edges to well-differentiated squamous epithelial cells. Some have deeply basophilic cytoplasm with perinuclear vacuolation and signs of asynchronous maturation of the nucleus and cytoplasm. Anisocytosis and anisokaryosis are moderate.

2 What are your differential diagnoses? Differential diagnoses include epithelial dysplasia and neoplasia (squamous cell carcinoma). Histopathology is required for a definitive diagnosis in the vast majority of the cases. Squamous cell carcinoma is a common finding in encrusted lesions on the pinnae and face of cats. In some cases, preneoplastic changes (actinic keratosis) may be identified.

Editors' note: Squamous cell carcinoma can vary from a very well-differentiated form to anaplastic, poorly differentiated forms. Cytologic features of squamous differentiation that may be found include keratinization, keratin 'pearls', intercellular bridges (cytoplasmic projections between adjacent cells), and/or polygonal cell shape with low N:C ratio. The presence of keratin precursors within squamous epithelial cells may be heralded by 'baby blue' cytoplasmic staining with Romanowsky stains or the presence of orangophilia with the Papanicolaou stain. In more anaplastic tumors the features that aid in recognition of squamous epithelial origin may be focal, infrequent, or absent. Squamous epithelial cells with spindloid or elongated appearance are also known as 'tadpole cells'. In well-differentiated tumors, nuclear features supportive of malignancy may be few, but the number of cells, location, smear pattern, and presence of an abnormal proliferation provide the background for interpretation of malignancy. Some squamous cell carcinomas may be ulcerated and include abundant neutrophilic and/or eosinophilic inflammation; the presence of inflammation does not ever rule out the possibility of concurrent neoplasia.

CASE 13

1 Describe the cells shown in the photomicrographs. The microphotographs are characterized by a clear background with frequent RBCs. There is a mixed population of nucleated cells, the majority being giant multinucleated cells and spindle-shaped mesenchymal cells; variable numbers of macrophages, occasional plasma cells, and small lymphocytes are also noted. Multinucleated giant cells have abundant basophilic cytoplasm, frequently forming multiple cytoplasmic tails. Nuclei are multiple, up to 20 per cell, round, with granular chromatin and prominent multiple small round nucleoli.

2 What are your differential diagnoses based on these cytologic findings? These findings are highly suggestive of a giant cell tumor of soft parts (GCTSP). A soft tissue sarcoma of other origin is also considered a possible differential diagnosis. GCTSP is a rare neoplasm, reported in several domestic species, including cats and horses (1% of all cutaneous equine neoplasms). It affects mostly adult animals, with no predisposition of sex and breed. These tumors usually appear as firm, raised, solitary and superficial masses attached to the superficial subcutaneous tissue. They have been described in several regions of the body, although there seems to be a predilection for the hindlimbs. Metastatic potential in horses appears to be very low and surgical excision with clean margins is considered to be curative. Local recurrence after incomplete surgical resection has been reported.

Surgical excision was performed with a defocused beam carbon dioxide laser under standing sedation and local anesthesia. The lesion was submitted for histopathologic examination, which confirmed the cytologic diagnosis. No recurrence was noted 6 months after surgery.

Further reading
Bush JM, Powers BE (2008) Equine giant cell tumour of soft parts: a series of 21 cases (2000–2007) *Journal of Veterinary Diagnostic Investigations* **20**:513–516.

CASE 14

1 Describe and classify the cells illustrated. Some cells are discrete, while others are in small groups with ill-defined margins. The cells vary in shape. Some are round; others have blunt cytoplasmic tails extending away from the nucleus (1, 2). These cytologic features are supportive of a mesenchymal origin.

2 What criteria of malignancy are present? Numerous criteria of malignancy are present. There is moderate to marked anisocytosis and anisokaryosis. There is a variable, but often high, N:C ratio. The nuclear chromatin is often stippled. There are several bi- and multinucleated cells. Nucleoli are prominent and frequently multiple (3).

3 Can you suggest a likely diagnosis? These cells are mesenchymal in origin. These atypical cytologic features, together with the clinical history of a distinct mass and the absence of inflammatory cells, are primarily suggestive of a mesenchymal neoplasia, likely a sarcoma. The type of sarcoma cannot be reliably determined from cytology and requires histopathology for further confirmation and characterization. A reactive fibroplasia (e.g. wound formation) is considered less likely, but cannot be ruled out on the sole basis of the cytology.

CASE 15

1 Identify the cell population present in the smear, and describe the most relevant characteristics. The samples are of high cellularity, containing a monolayer of cohesive cells arranged in variably sized sheets and clusters with acinar and palisading patterns. Cells are monomorphic, round to polygonal, often with poorly defined cytoplasmic borders. The cytoplasm is moderate, with some cells containing few to moderate, clear, round vacuoles. Nuclei are uniform and round, with fine chromatin and small round nucleoli (**15a**). Overall, cellular atypia is slight. In some areas the N:C ratio is low, and the cells show more distinct cytoplasmic borders (**15b**).

2 What differential diagnoses would you consider for an ovarian mass? Differential diagnoses for a solid ovarian mass include tumors of various origin: epithelial (e.g. adenoma, adenocarcinoma), gonadostromal (e.g. granulosa cell tumor, luteoma, thecoma), germ cell (e.g. dysgerminoma, teratoma, embryonal carcinoma), and mesenchymal (.g. leiomyoma).

3 What is your final interpretation? Based on the cellular arrangement, epithelial or gonadostromal tumors are the most likely differentials. The acinar arrangement and the cell vacuolation are both supportive of a steroid secreting origin, which is also the likely cause of the clinical signs (e.g. hyperoestrogenism). The presence of acinar structures containing amorphous eosinophilic material (**15c**, arrow) are referred to in human cytologic samples as Call–Exner bodies, and are considered strongly suggestive of a granulosa cell tumor.

Further reading
Bertazzolo W, Dell'Orco M, Bonfanti U *et al.* (2004) Cytological features of canine ovarian tumors: a retrospective study on 19 cases. *Journal of Small Animal Practice* **45:** 539–545.

CASE 16
Identify the exogenous and possible foreign body material in this photomicrograph (16; Wright–Giemsa, ×50 oil). The photomicrograph shows starch grains within blood alongside a neoplastic mesenchymal population and matrical material (on the right side). The former are contaminants sticking to the slide from 'powdered' gloves worn during sampling. Starch grains are colorless to pale yellow–green, and refractile, with a central cruciate structure.

CASE 17
1 Describe the cells present. There is moderate pleomorphism and anisokaryosis of the cells in **17b**. The cells in **17a** are arranged in an acinar or ductal configuration around a central lumen. Many cells have a high N:C ratio, with a coarse nuclear chromatin pattern and prominent nucleoli. Some of these nucleoli are macronucleoli (>5μm diameter).
2 What is the cell line of origin of these cells? The adherent nature and cohesiveness of these cells indicates an epithelial origin. The nuclei in **17a** are at the periphery of the cells, indicating an acinar or ductal formation, which, in turn, suggests a tumor of secretory or glandular tissue.
3 Are there features present that suggest malignancy? Pleomorphism, anisokaryosis, increased N:C ratio, a coarse chromatin pattern, macronucleoli, and variation in nucleolar size and shape are all criteria of malignancy. Given the presence of these criteria, the probable glandular origin, and the site of the lesion, these features most likely reflect a ceruminous gland adenocarcinoma. Histologic evaluation confirmed a ceruminous gland adenocarcinoma with lymphatic spread.

Editors' note: Ceruminous gland tumors are more frequent in cats than in dogs. They are often associated with a history of chronic irritation and infection.

Hyperplasia and adenomas may be difficult to differentiate cytologically and clinically. Adenocarcinomas are diagnosed based on features of malignancy. Adenocarcinomas are locally invasive and may metastasize to regional lymph nodes. Occasionally, more distant metastases are identified.

CASE 18

1 Describe the cells shown in the photomicrographs. The photomicrographs show a cluster of large nucleated cells in a background of RBCs. These cells appear large, with abundant lightly basophilic cytoplasm and, occasionally, fringed cytoplasmic borders. Nuclei are round, paracentral, with coarse granular chromatin, and contain up to three, prominent, round nucleoli. Anisocytosis and anisokaryosis are moderate. Binucleated and multinucleated elements are also seen.

2 What are your differential diagnoses based on these cytologic findings, and what additional tests would you recommend? Given the clinical history and the amount of atypia that is present, malignancy is the primary concern. Differentials should include epithelial or mesothelial origin. Sometimes a reactive mesothelial proliferation will mimic malignancy, but the degree of atypia and presence of a well-defined mass are more in favor of a malignancy. Histopathology and immunohistochemistry are needed to determine the most definitive diagnosis. Mesothelial cells frequently (but not always) show co-expression of cytokeratin and vimentin. However, some visceral neoplasms of epithelial origin may also show co-expression of epithelial and mesenchymal markers (e.g. renal carcinoma, pulmonary carcinoma, Sertoli cell tumor, thyroid tumors). The clinical history and imaging findings may be very helpful in the diagnostic process, especially when there is evidence of a primary mass. In this case the absence of other masses/lesions, the histologic and immunohistochemical findings (co-expression of cytokeratin/vimentin) (18c, d; cytokeratin and vimentin, respectively, ×40)

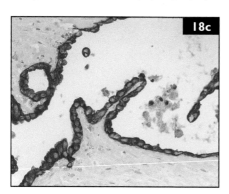
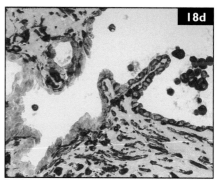

were considered compatible with an epithelioid mesothelioma. The cat recovered from the general anesthesia, although clinical signs persisted. NSAIDs and intracavitary platinum-based chemotherapy were proposed to the owners. After 2 weeks of prolonged anorexia, lethargy, and weight loss, the owners elected for euthanasia.

Further reading
Bacci B, Morandi F, De Meo M *et al.* (2006) Ten cases of feline mesothelioma: an immunhistochemical and ultrastructural study. *Journal of Comparative Pathology* 134:347–354.

CASE 19

1 Describe the cytologic features of the nucleated cells. There is a monomorphic population of nucleated cells characterized by moderate amounts of basophilic cytoplasm. The cytoplasm contains small clear vacuoles and has poorly distinct cytoplasmic borders. Nuclei are paracentrally located, with granular chromatin and indistinct nucleoli.

2 What is the likely origin/type of these cells? These cells appear neuroendocrine in origin and do not demonstrate significant criteria of malignancy.

3 Based on this group of cells, what diagnosis would you make in this case? The cytologic diagnosis is adrenocortical hyperplasia/neoplasia. Histopathology confirmed an adrenocortical adenoma. In one report of 18 cases of hyperadrenocorticism, 14 cats were diagnosed with pituitary-dependent hyperadrenocorticism and four cats with a unilateral adrenocortical tumor (2 adrenocortical carcinomas, 2 adrenal adenomas).

Editors' note: The identification of hyperadrenocorticism in this case was well supported by other laboratory data and the localization of a distinct mass in the right adrenal gland was supportive of a tumor. In other cases the presence of an intra-abdominal mass may be the initial observation and ultrasound-guided fine needle aspiration may be the initial avenue of investigation. In those cases the organ or cell type of origin of the mass may not be clinically apparent. Some differences in the appearance of adrenal mass aspirates and impression smears should be kept in mind. In this case an impression smear shows primarily intact cells with the classic vacuolated appearance that is typical of an adrenocortical origin. Aspirates from adrenal masses are reported to more commonly contain large numbers of nuclei that have been stripped of cytoplasm or which appear in a background of lightly basophilic cytoplasm with indistinct borders. This appearance is typical of neuroendocrine neoplasia. Intact cells similar to the ones illustrated in this case may also be present in variable numbers. If marked anaplasia or pleomorphic features consistent with malignancy are present, a diagnosis of a malignant neoplasia is possible. However, well-differentiated carcinomas may be difficult to distinguish from adenomas and additional histologic evaluation and clinical investigation of possible metastasis may be needed to help distinguish adrenocortical adenomas from well-differentiated carcinomas.

Further reading
Bertazzolo W, Didier M, Gelain ME *et al.* (2014) Accuracy of cytology in distinguishing adrenocortical tumors from pheochromocytoma in companion animals. *Veterinary Clinical Pathology* **43(3):**453–459.
Duesberg C, Petersen ME (1997) Adrenal disorders in cats. *Veterinary Clinics of North America: Small Animal Practice* **27(2):**321–347.

CASE 20

1 Describe the findings seen in the photomicrograph. The photomicrograph shows a mixed population of nucleated cells, the majority being eosinophils, with a lower percentage of reactive foamy macrophages and a few lymphocytes. There is evidence of a yeast form with a distinctive nonstaining, thick, mucoid capsule surrounding a granular basophilic internal structure, compatible with *Cryptococcus* (indicated by the arrow).

2 What is your interpretation based on these cytologic findings? These findings are indicative of a moderate, mixed, mostly eosinophilic pleocytosis associated with fungal infection with *Cryptococcus*. Eosinophilic pleocytosis in CSF of dogs is associated with infectious diseases (including protozoa, parasites, fungi, distemper virus, rabies) hypersensitivity reactions, neoplastic processes, and steroid-responsive eosinophilic meningitis; it may be part of a nonspecific acute inflammatory response or may be idiopathic.

Cryptococcus infection in dogs frequently presents as a disseminated disease with central nervous system and/or ocular involvement. Serologic and molecular methods may be helpful when the organism is not observed on cytology.

Despite appropriate therapy, the dog continued to deteriorate, developed intracranial neurologic signs, and was euthanized 3 weeks after the diagnosis.

CASE 21

1 Identify the etiologic agent in this exudative effusion, with precise reference to the exact stage of its life cycle as seen in the photomicrographs. Intracellular protozoon consistent with *Toxoplasma gondii*. Stage: tachyzoites, multiplying within macrophages and neutrophils (insert lower right corner, **21b**).

Answers

2 What other laboratory tests would you like to use to support your cytologic suspicion? Serology.

3 Given the following laboratory results, what can you determine about the kinetics of *Toxoplasma gondii* from these values: IgM – ELISA ~ 1:256; IgG – ELISA ~ 1:64? IgM antibodies can identify early infection at 1–2 weeks post exposure. They peak at 3–6 weeks and usually drop to negative at 12 weeks post exposure. Caution: some cats can have sporadic low IgM ELISA titers for up to one year post exposure. IgG antibodies develop at approximately 2 weeks post infection and can remain high for several years to the life of the cat. Based on the high IgM titer and presence of IgG, this patient has an active, progressing to established *T. gondii* infection. A diagnosis of active infection can also be made by a four-fold increase in serial IgG tests 2–3 weeks apart.

4 Toxoplasmosis is a potential zoonotic risk. Are cat owners and veterinarians at significantly higher risk than the general population of acquiring *T. gondii* infection? No. Minimizing risk does not have to include prevention of exposure to cats but must prevent exposure to oocysts (particularly sporulated oocysts). Therefore, pregnant women and immunocompromised individuals should not change cat litter boxes, should wear gloves when gardening, and should maintain extra hygiene when working with food products, particularly raw meat. Only sporulated oocysts are infective; therefore, litter must be changed daily and, given the fastidious grooming habits of cats, they are unlikely to be a risk since they do not have sporulated oocysts on their fur.

5 Are seropositive cats a risk for pregnant women or immunocompromised individuals? No. Most seropositive cats have completed the oocyst shedding period and are unlikely to repeat shedding (for up to 6 years).

CASE 22

1 What are the principles of quality assurance in veterinary cytology, and how can diagnostic accuracy be determined in veterinary cytology? Laboratory performance and quality of the results can be affected by preanalytical, analytical, and postanalytical factors. Documentation of specific policies, monitoring, and corrective actions should be established for all areas of the laboratory by quality assurance programs. In veterinary cytology, specimen collection, handling, delivery, and identification are preanalytical factors that should be addressed and standardized. The cytologist has an essential role in offering educational support to clients and in reducing the number of inadequate specimens submitted.

Standard preparations, fixation, and staining procedures of specimens are analytical factors addressed by internal nonstatistical quality control programs; these can vary between individual laboratories according to the techniques used and cytologist preferences. Diagnostic accuracy should be determined through follow-up procedures. This consists of comparison of findings with histologic or additional cytologic specimens, information about clinical progress of the patient, and other diagnostic tests in order to assess correlation of the results. When discrepancies between results are noted, specimen review is indicated to determine if there are features that have been overlooked or misinterpreted.

Finally, the accuracy of results can be affected by postanalytical factors. A standard format for the reports, which should be easily understood and have appropriate explanations, is the cytologist's responsibility. Attribution of the interpretation to the correct animal and reporting of the results to the correct clinician in a timely manner are other aspects of the postanalytic process.

Further reading
Gunn-Christie RG, Flatland B, Friedrichs KR *et al.*; American Society for Veterinary Clinical Pathology (ASVCP) (2012) ASVCP quality assurance guidelines: control of preanalytical, analytical, and postanalytical factors for urinalysis, cytology, and clinical chemistry in veterinary laboratories. *Veterinary Clinical Pathology* 41(1):18–26.

CASE 23

1 Describe the cells shown in the photomicrographs. There are epithelioid or neuroendocrine cells arranged in cohesive groups with more circular acinoid arrangements. These cells have cuboidal to coalescent, moderately basophilic cytoplasm, which is occasionally discretely vacuolated. While not markedly pleomorphic, more than 3–5 features of malignancy are still seen with irregular arrangements showing cellular crowding, nuclei with variably coarse to clumped and hyperchromatic chromatin within a thickened nuclear membrane, variable nuclear size (moderate anisokaryosis), cellular fragmentation, and individualization.

2 What is your interpretation of these findings? The cytologic features are consistent with an insulinoma or endocrine pancreatic neoplasia. The atypical features support malignancy. Metastatic proliferation is commonly seen, although features of malignancy are often not marked. While not shown here, the cells can also be variably but more discretely vacuolated nuclei with a variably prominent nucleolus.

CASE 24

1 Describe the cells shown in the photomicrograph. The photomicrograph shows a monomorphic population of discrete round cells, characterized by moderate amounts of granular basophilic cytoplasm, and variable numbers of clear distinct intracytoplasmic vacuoles, occasionally arranged along the cytoplasmic boundary. Nuclei are round, central to paracentral, with coarse chromatin and usually a single, prominent, round nucleolus. Anisocytosis and anisokaryosis are moderate.

2 What is your diagnosis based on these cytologic findings? These cytologic features, together with the clinical history/findings, are indicative of a round cell tumor, and more specifically of a transmissible venereal tumor (TVT). TVT is a histiocytic tumor of the external genitalia, described in the dog and other canines living in temperate climates. Preferred locations include external genitalia and all the mucous membranes associated with sexual contact. In this specific case, TVT was confirmed on histopathology (incisional biopsy). The lesion underwent complete regression after 4 weekly doses of vincristine.

CASE 25

1 Describe the cells represented in the smears. A mixed population of macrophages with a foamy cytoplasm and small lymphocytes are seen in 25a. At high magnification (25b) the foamy aspect of the cytoplasm of the macrophages is shown to be due to the presence of numerous clear, slender, elongated intracytoplasmic inclusions. The positive Ziehl–Neelsen-stained smear (25c) shows numerous red acid-fast bacilli.

2 What is your interpretation, and what are the differential diagnoses? Diagnosis: mycobacteriosis (*Mycobacterium lepraemurium*). Differential diagnosis: none.

CASE 26

1 Describe the cytologic findings, and give your cytologic interpretation. There are a few small clusters of well-differentiated hepatocytes admixed with abundant eosinophilic dense amorphous material, suggestive of amyloid. Deposition of amyloid occurs as a consequence of long-standing inflammatory processes and/ or tissue destruction, which both may lead to liver production of its precursor, the acute phase protein serum amyloid A. Deposition may occur in several organs, including kidney, spleen, and liver. Clinical signs may vary, depending on which organ is being affected, the amount of amyloid that is deposited, and the reaction of the organ to the amyloid deposition. In some cases, amyloidosis may result in organ failure.

2 What additional tests might be useful in order to confirm the diagnosis? Congo Red stain is a histochemical stain that helps to confirm the deposition of amyloid, which will appear orange/red under standard light microscopy and apple-green under polarized light.

CASE 27

1 Identify the cells or structures labeled 1, 2, 3, and 4 in 27a and 27b, and state their significance in the context of a bronchoalveolar lavage. 1 = columnar ciliated respiratory epithelial cells (confirms that the sample successfully obtained cells representative of the respiratory tract as far distally as the major airways [trachea, bronchi]; 2 = superficial squamous epithelial cell (indicates that there is a degree of oral contamination); 3 = the bacteria on the surface of the squamous epithelial cells, which are *Simonsiella* species; these are normal inhabitants of the oral pharynx and also indicate that the wash is contaminated; 4 = Curschmann's spirals (inspissated mucus).

2 Interpret the pathologic process seen in 27c. Marked, mixed, septic, predominantly eosinophilic inflammation.

3 How do you know that the bacteria present in this wash are likely to be significant? Bacteria are present within lysosomes, in the cytoplasm of eosinophils that have phagocytosed them.

4 Are eosinophils more or less effective at phagocytosing and killing bacteria than neutrophils? Less effective. Although eosinophils have receptors that allow them to phagocytose bacteria, they have a lower density of complement receptors than neutrophils and, despite high levels of peroxidase activity, oxidative responses and H_2O_2 than neutrophils involved in the killing process of bacteria, they lack several bactericidal substances (lactoferrin and phagocytin) and their cationic proteins have weak or no bactericidal or inflammatory properties.

Editors' note: Curschmann's spirals are associated with conditions characterized by chronic and excessive production of mucus. They may occur in respiratory and reproductive cytology specimens and, in humans, have been reported in specimens from body cavity (pleural and peritoneal) fluids.

Superficial squamous epithelial cells, with or without bacteria, in respiratory cytology specimens are the result of oropharyngeal contamination in most cases. The amount of contamination may vary but, with experienced and careful collectors, is usually low.

Squamous metaplasia may occur in the respiratory system in response to chronic irritation. In this condition the columnar to cuboidal epithelium of the airways is replaced by stratified, flattened epithelium. It is usually a focal to focally extensive change. It is thought to represent an attempt at repair and protection from chronic irritation but may, in fact, lead to a nonfunctional and nonprotective epithelium that does not have normal secretion or mucociliary apparatus function. The development of squamous metaplasia is preceded by proliferation of reserve or basal cells, a change that may be visible as increased thickness and numbers of small, uniform, tightly cohesive cells with scant cytoplasm in tissue fragments. As these cells mature and differentiate, they resemble maturing squamous epithelium but are smaller and have a higher N:C ratio. There may be an increase in granularity of chromatin and hyperchromasia and nucleoli may be present with increasing atypia and progression to dysplasia. In human studies, squamous metaplasia and dysplasia have been found to antedate the appearance of carcinoma of the lung. Severe dysplasia may mimic carcinoma or represent so-called bronchial intraepithelial neoplasia that may, in some cases, progress to invasive cancer. These changes have not been studied in detail in dogs to see if the same potential biological behavior and progression are present. However, squamous metaplasia has been recognized in respiratory cytology specimens from dogs and horses and is interpreted to represent a response to marked, chronic irritation.

Further reading
Baker R, Lumsden JH (2000) *Color Atlas of Cytology of the Dog and Cat*, 1st edn. Mosby, St. Louis, pp. 23–29.
Cotran RS, Kumar V, Collins T (1999) (eds) *Robbins Pathologic Basis of Disease*, 6th edn. WB Saunders, Philadelphia, p. 196.
Feldman BF, Zinkl JG, Jain NC (2000) *Schalm's Veterinary Hematology*, 5th edn. Lippincott Williams and Wilkins, Philadelphia, p. 304.
Jain NC (1993) *Essentials of Veterinary Hematology*. Lee & Febiger, Philadelphia, p. 253.

CASE 28
1 Describe the structure shown in the smear. There is a large blue-staining structure containing multiple, oval, elongated nuclei. Nucleoli are not recognized. In some areas, multiple parallel striations or 'stripes' are seen perpendicular to the long axis of the structure.
2 What is your interpretation? This structure is a striated (skeletal) muscle fragment.
3 What are your differential diagnoses? Possible differentials include spurious aspiration of muscle and rhabdomyoma.

CASE 29
1 What is the most important feature in this liver aspirate? In some areas, you can appreciate dark ribbons of inspissated bile that form casts within the biliary canaliculi (indicated by the arrows) that course between hepatocytes (extracytoplasmic cholestasis); hepatocytes show mild cytoplasmic rarefaction and contain variable numbers of poorly defined clear cytoplasmic vacuoles, supportive of mild cytoplasmic degeneration, likely due to microvesicular steatosis (more marked in other areas of the smear). The presence of small numbers of neutrophils and small lymphocytes (subjectively more than expected for this degree of blood

contamination) may suggest mild concurrent inflammation, although no leukocytes are seen in close association with the hepatocytes. Extracytoplasmic cholestasis is secondary to obstruction of the biliary outflow; possible differentials for this may include stones in the gallbladder or in biliary ducts, mucinous hyperplasia of the gallbladder, severe inflammation of the biliary ducts, or primary or secondary hepatic neoplasms.

2 Based on all these findings, what is the most likely cause for this condition?
Inflammation. Increased values of haptoglobin and C reactive protein suggest the presence of acute inflammation, and are further supported by the increased number of circulating toxic neutrophils and monocytes. Abdominal ultrasound findings suggested an inflammatory process within the gallbladder wall; surgical procedures revealed the presence of stones in the gallbladder, with inflammation and focal necrosis.

CASE 30
1 Identify the organism. *Blastomyces dermatitidis*.
2 What is the primary morphologic finding used to identify this organism?
Blastomyces dermatitidis is characterized by a prominent cell wall with no evidence of endosporulation and broad-based budding. The nonbudding forms can be easily confused with small spherules of *Coccidioides* species. While *Coccidioides* spherules can be as large as 120 microns, the yeast forms of *Blastomyces dermatitidis* are usually no larger than 15 microns. While the geographic distribution of the two fungi does not overlap, both diseases should be considered if there has been travel to an endemic area. Finding a budding form of *Blastomyces dermatitidis* or a large endosporulating spherule in the case of *Coccidioides* will definitively differentiate the two infectious agents. Since there is minimal cross-reactivity between the agar gel immunodiffusion serologic tests for these two organisms, serology can assist is differentiating the two fungi if there are no defining characteristics found in the cytologic preparations.

Further reading
Dial SM (2007) Fungal diagnostics: current techniques and future trends. *Veterinary Clinics of North America: Small Animal Practice* 37:373–392.

CASE 31
1 Describe your findings. There are large numbers of keratin bars and frequent broad-based budding structures resembling the sole of a shoe, most compatible with yeast. The most likely differential is *Malassezia pachydermatis* (also known as *Malassezia canis*).

Answers

2 **How do you decide whether yeasts are significant or not?** A diagnosis of mycotic otitis externa is supported by the identification of >10 organisms per ×40 objective or >4 organisms per oil immersion field. *Malassezia* is found three times more frequently in otitic ears than in normal ears.

3 **By what proposed theories does *Malassezia* cause otitis?** The inflammation may be due to the by-products of lipid/*Malassezia* interaction (e.g. formation of peroxides) or type I hypersensitivity reaction to *Malassezia* and its by-products.

4 **What special stains can be used to demonstrate *Malassezia*, and what are the staining characteristics with these stains?** Gram stain: basophilic color; PAS stain: PAS-positive, bright magenta color.

Further reading

Ettinger SJ, Feldman EC (2010) *Textbook of Veterinary Internal Medicine*, 7th edn. WB Saunders, Philadelphia.

Rausch FD, Skinner GW (1978) Incidence and treatment of budding yeast in canine otitis externa. *Modern Veterinary Practice* 53:914–915

Scott DW (1980) External ear disorders. *Journal of the American Animal Hospital Association* 16:426–433.

CASE 32

1 **What processes are indicated in the photomicrographs?** Both photomicrographs show variably intact and degenerating cellular material within neutrophils and macrophages. There is a multinucleated giant macrophage with dense clear white cytoplasmic vacuoles (**32a**) and two clumps of notched rectangular colorless crystalline clefts (**32b**). The vacuoles and crystals are consistent with fat/lipid and cholesterol, indicating phagocytosis and deposition/degradation. The yellow material otherwise is likely bilirubin and supports previous hemorrhage.

2 **What is your final interpretation?** With the pyogranulomatous inflammation, these findings are compatible with a xanthoma. These lesions can be seen with underlying lipid dysmetabolism (such as hyperlipidemia, diabetes mellitus, hypothyroidism, and hyperadrenocorticism), but their exact etiology is unclear. In contrast, subcutaneous steatitis (panniculitis) is typically neither pyogranulomatous nor a distinct cutaneous mass. Xanthomas are more commonly observed in the subcutis of the head, ears, and inguinum or in internal organs.

CASE 33

1 **What cells are present?** Apart from RBCs, there is a single population of pleomorphic spindloid cells. These vary from round to spindle shaped, and they have moderate amounts of basophilic cytoplasm with indefinite boundaries.

Nuclei are round to fusiform with clumped chromatin and one to two nucleoli. The findings are indicative of mesenchymal proliferation, likely neoplastic.

2 What is your interpretation? Mesenchymal proliferation. Differential diagnoses include reactive fibroplasia, sarcoid, and soft tissue sarcoma. A fibrosarcoma was confirmed on postmortem examination.

Editors' note: The main differential diagnoses that should be considered for spindle cell tumors/mesenchymal tumors in horses include fibroma, fibrosarcoma, and equine sarcoid. Other types of mesenchymal tumors are very uncommon. It may be difficult or impossible to differentiate these tumors based on cytologic features alone. Consideration of the clinical appearance and location may be helpful, but definitive diagnosis usually requires histologic evaluation.

CASE 34

1 Describe the cytologic findings of these photomicrographs. On a background containing large numbers of RBCs, there are several clusters of cohesive cells, organized in a papillary pattern. Cells are mostly large, with a low N:C ratio. The cytoplasm is abundant, finely granular, pinkish to blue, with defined borders. Nuclei are centrally located, oval to round, with granular chromatin and a prominent single, round nucleolus. These cells are epithelial in origin and are part of some intradermal modified sebaceous glands (perianal glands), commonly observed in the perianal region in dogs. Because of their resemblance to hepatocytes, these cells are also referred as 'hepatoid'. The few small cells pointed to by the arrow are cuboidal reserve cells. These may be normally present in low numbers in sebaceous adenomas. They appear as small basaloid cells, with small, condensed nuclei, frequently arranged in rows.

2 What is your interpretation? These findings are supportive of a perianal gland tumor. Adenomas and well-differentiated carcinomas cannot be differentiated on the sole basis of the cytology, since they may appear similar. However, adenoma is more common and is mostly associated with intact male dogs (androgen dependency), whereas the malignant counterpart of this tumor is less frequently encountered.

CASE 35

1 Describe the cytologic features seen in the photomicrographs, and provide a general description. The aspirate harvested large numbers of nucleated cells, arranged in clusters or sheets, occasionally forming acinar structures and palisades. These cells, likely epithelial in origin, have indistinct cytoplasmic borders and appear as free nuclei embedded in a background of greyish–blue cytoplasm. Nuclei are round to oval, with fine granular chromatin, small indistinct nucleoli, and minimal features of atypia, including mild anisokaryosis. Extracellular amorphous pink material (consistent with colloid) is sometimes noted and is associated with the clusters.

The presence of colloid, together with the nuclei within a background of poorly defined cytoplasm, are both cytologic features commonly observed in thyroid aspirates.

2 What is your interpretation, and what further investigations would you recommend? Thyroid neoplasia, likely thyroid follicular carcinoma. Approximately 90–95% of clinically apparent canine thyroid tumors are adenocarcinomas and have a malignant behavior (high invasiveness and metastatic tendency). Well-differentiated forms showing only mild cytologic features of atypia are commonly observed. Therefore, any time a canine mass is identified as thyroid in origin, it should be considered as a probable carcinoma until histopathologic confirmation is obtained. Thyroid neoplasms are commonly highly vascularized and locally invasive, making incisional or excisional biopsies complicated.

When thyroid neoplasia is present, measurement of thyroid hormones may be considered, although in dogs hypersecretion of thyroid hormones in association with a thyroid tumor is uncommon and may involve only 10% of cases.

Editors' note: It may be difficult to determine if the nuclei within poorly defined cytoplasm are sufficient for a cytologic diagnosis or represent a poorly preserved specimen of other origin that is unsuitable for interpretation. Knowledge of the species, site of the tumor, and careful examination of the cell preservation should be undertaken to make this judgment. Well-differentiated forms of some malignant tumors (e.g. thyroid carcinoma, hepatocellular carcinoma, soft tissue sarcoma) frequently do not show significant cytologic features of malignancy, and may appear cytologically similar to their benign counterparts. Malignancy can be suspected from the clinical behavior (e.g. rapid growth, high metastatic rate), knowledge of the site, and type of tumor suspected, and commonly requires histopathology for definitive confirmation.

CASE 36

1 What cells are present? The smear contains neutrophils and cell debris (not seen in the picture), but there are also clusters of pleomorphic epithelial cells. These vary from benign keratinized mature squames (deep blue structure, top left of **36b**, partially out of the field) to epithelial cells with abundant basophilic cytoplasm, angular cytoplasmic borders, and frequent clear punctate vacuoles, occasionally perinuclear. Some of these cells are binucleated; the nuclei have coarse granular chromatin and prominent round nucleoli. Anisocytosis and anisokaryosis are moderate.

2 What is the cytologic interpretation? Squamous cell carcinoma. The eyelid is a relatively common site for this tumor in the cow. The presence of neutrophils (not seen in the picture) indicates concurrent inflammation, which is likely secondary to the underlying neoplasia and due to the ulcerative nature of the lesion.

CASE 37

1 Describe the features shown. There is a hair root and shaft base showing loss of cortical and medullary distinction due to long chains of refractile circular arthrospores.

2 What is your interpretation of these findings? These findings are indicative of dermatophytosis. While many species of dermatophytes are fluorescent under UV light, *Microsporum canis* is not. Microscopy on hair plucks or deep skin scrapes that include capillary ooze and fresh blood should be used for diagnosis, especially with ectoparasites such as *Demodex*. Use of Calcofluor-White stain can aid detection of extracuticular spores under fluorescent light, but is less specific.

CASE 38

1 What cell types are present in the photomicrographs? There are a few to a moderate number of neutrophils and a moderate number of macrophages in **38a**. There are three siderophages (macrophages containing large clumps of green pigment) in the upper central portion of the figure. There is a small amount of thin mucus in the background, with many macrophages in **38b**. Three siderophages are present.

2 What differences do you notice in the siderophages shown in these photomicrographs? The siderophages in **38a** contain larger, more darkly stained clumps of hemosiderin compared with the siderophages in **38b**. The siderophages in **38b** contain finer, more lightly stained granules of hemosiderin. The finer, more lightly stained siderophages have been designated as 'early siderophages' and usually occur between three and 14 days following blood instillation or observation of bleeding endoscopically. The siderophages containing larger, more darkly stained clumps of hemosiderin are termed 'aged siderophages' and are observed more than 14 days following blood instillation or endoscopic hemorrhage.

The ease with which hemosiderin is recognized in the Papanicolaou-stained smears is an advantage of this stain over Romanowsky stains for equine respiratory specimens. A Perl's Prussian Blue stain can be applied directly over the Papanicolaou-stained preparation if additional confirmation of the presence of iron is desired. **38c** (Perl's Prussian Blue, ×16) shows several macrophages in an equine tracheal washing with blue, granular cytoplasmic material confirmatory of iron and the presence of hemosiderin. **38d** (Perl's Prussian Blue, ×25) shows a diffusely stained, pale blue macrophage with some orange erythrocytes in the background of a tracheal washing. In some specimens these diffusely stained, iron-positive cells can be detected in cells without the presence of recognizable hemosiderin granules. Their significance is not certain but they are only consistently found in specimens from horses with confirmed pulmonary hemorrhage.

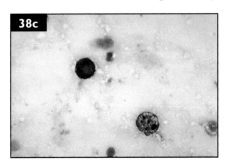

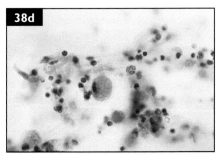

3 What is your interpretation of the cytologic findings? The simultaneous appearance of 'early siderophages' and 'aged siderophages' in a respiratory cytology specimen supports the presence of hemorrhage on more than one occasion. Other features of the smear (not all of which are illustrated) include abundant thin mucus, active macrophages, few to moderate number of neutrophils, and focal and slight atypia of columnar and cuboidal epithelial cells consistent with bronchitis and bronchiolitis. No eosinophils were seen. This combination of cellular and noncellular features is consistent with the pattern of exercise-induced pulmonary hemorrhage.

Further reading
Cian F, Monti P, Durham A (2015) Cytology of the lower respiratory tract in horses: an updated review. *Equine Veterinary Education* **27**(10):544–553.
Freeman KP, Roszel JF (1997) Patterns in equine respiratory cytology specimens associated with respiratory conditions of noninfectious or unknown etiology. *Compendium on Continuing Education for the Practicing Veterinarian* **19**(6):755–763, 783.
Roszel JF, Freeman KP, Slusher SH *et al.* (1988) Siderophages in pulmonary cytology specimens from racing and nonracing horses. *Proceedings of the 33rd Convention of the American Association of Equine Practitioners*, New Orleans, pp. 321–329.
Step DL, Freeman KP, Gleed R, Hackett R (1991) Cytological and endoscopic findings after intrapulmonary blood inoculation in horses. *Journal of Equine Veterinary Science* **119**(6):340–345.

CASE 39

1 Describe the features shown in the photomicrographs. There is a population of nucleated cells, likely myoepithelial in origin, with cells cohesive but slender and elongated. Peripherally there are swirls and strands or fragmenting sheets. Individual cells show moderate anisocytosis and anisokaryosis. Their nuclei are circular to oval or irregular, with variably coarse chromatin and indistinct, variably sized nucleoli. Their cytoplasm is pale to medium blue and demarcated to wispy. Intercellular strands of eosinophilic fibrillary or hyalinized material also are seen (stroma and scirrhous reaction). These groups show cellular crowding and more irregular arrangements. Neither mastitis nor significant ectasia/dilation is evident.
2 What is your interpretation of these findings? This is a mammary carcinoma, likely complex rather than simple. No convincing mixed mesenchymal elements are seen.

Editors' note: Diagnosing carcinomas and discriminating between simple and complex epithelial mammary neoplasia is controversial. Splitting and grading is potentially possible, as in histopathology, but currently there are no clear, widely accepted criteria based on the cytopathologic features alone.

CASE 40

1 What cells are present? There are a few RBCs but nearly all the nucleated cells are from a single population of pleomorphic cells. They are round to spindle shaped and there is moderate anisocytosis and anisokaryosis. Nuclei are round to oval, with coarse granular chromatin and prominent round nucleoli. Cytoplasm is basophilic and borders are indistinct. A few cells (see cell at far right in **40b**) contain dark-greenish granules, which are consistent with melanin.
2 What is your interpretation? Melanoma.

Editors' note: Poorly differentiated, amelanotic, or poorly melanotic melanomas are 'great pretenders' and may have features that suggest epithelial and/or mesenchymal origin cytologically. As in this case, diligent searching may result in the identification of a few cells with small numbers of melanin granules or blue–green to black material consistent with melanin. In other cases, melanoma may be suspected but melanin not demonstrated.

CASE 41

1 Describe the cytologic findings and give your cytologic interpretation. There are high numbers of RBCs observed in the background, together with a few platelet clumps (1), small numbers of lymphocytes and neutrophils, likely blood derived, and a small group of mesenchymal spindle cells, likely fibroblasts (2). A microfilaria (larval form of the tissue filarial nematode) is also present in the bottom right of the picture (3). Differential diagnosis includes a granuloma with microfilaria infection. The presence of microfilaria may also be the result of blood contamination in a dog with microfilaremia.

2 What additional tests might be useful to confirm the diagnosis? Additional investigations may include histopathology of the mass and further testing to characterize the microfilaria, including the modified Knott's test, serology, and PCR testing. There are morphologic criteria to help differentiate between microfilaria of *Dirofilaria* or *Dipetolema*, which are common microfilaria in dogs. An infection by *Dirofilaria repens* was confirmed in this case. Histopathologic diagnosis of the mass revealed a cutaneous hemangioma; no microfilaria or adult worms in the lesion were observed. Therefore, the presence of the microfilaria was likely the result microfilaremia with blood contamination during the aspiration of the mass.

Further reading
Bredal WP, Gjerde B, Eberhard ML *et al.* (1998) Adult *Dirofilaria repens* in a subcutaneous granuloma on the chest of a dog. *Journal of Small Animal Practice* **39**:595–597.

CASE 42

1 Identify the cell population present in the smear, and describe the most relevant characteristics. The samples have adequate cellularity and preservation and contain abundant amorphous basophilic granular material on the background, admixed with clear empty spaces (most likely lipid droplets) and a few adipocytes. Variable numbers of inflammatory cells are seen throughout the smear, the majority being nondegenerate neutrophils, and a small percentage of macrophages (**42a**). At higher magnification, some macrophages contain vacuolated cytoplasm with variable amounts of phagocytosed amorphous yellow material (**42b**).

2 What is your final interpretation? The described microscopic features are consistent with a neutrophilic and macrophagic inflammation of the panniculus (panniculitis/steatitis) with possible steatonecrosis. The yellow intracytoplasmic material may represent a nonspecific finding; however, an exogenous substance, such as drugs injected in the subcutaneous area after surgery, is another possible consideration.

Editors' note: This cytologic appearance is also typical of injection site reactions. In the interscapular region this is an important differential diagnosis and review of the history to determine if an injection may have been given at this location is recommended.

CASE 43

1 Describe the features illustrated. The low-power photomicrograph indicates a very highly cellular sample with large numbers of neutrophils contained within copious amounts of mucinous material. Many of the neutrophils are degenerate and smeared. Within this mix are a number of basophilic 'fluffy' particles. The high-power photomicrograph shows one of the fluffy particles in greater detail. The particle is composed of numerous basophilic filamentous rod-shaped organisms, whose terminal portions in some cases have become club shaped. The neutrophils present show karyorhexis and karyolysis.

2 What is your interpretation of these findings? These findings indicate a severe septic neutrophilic inflammation. The organisms have the typical appearance of either *Actinomyces* or *Nocardia* species in their 'ray fungi' form, as seen in actinomycosis/nocardiosis. Culture is necessary for diagnosis of the specific type and samples should be obtained anaerobically. The clubbed ends are gelatinous sheaths containing deposits of calcium phosphate.

3 What other conditions is this organism associated with? *Actinomyces* species are gram-positive, microaerophilic to anaerobic, non-acid-fast rods that show occasional branching. *Nocardia* species are gram positive but variably positive to acid-fast stain. Infection commonly starts by traumatic introduction of the pathogen into the skin (penetrating wounds), leading to dermatitis, cellulitis, and cutaneous nodules. Hematogenous dissemination may follow and cause abscesses to internal organs, pleuritis/peritonitis, and pyothrorax.

CASE 44

1 Describe the cells seen in the smear. What is your interpretation? A population of large pleomorphic oval to spindle-shaped cells are the predominant cell type in this lymph node aspirate. They are generally scattered individually but in some areas there appears to be intercellular cohesion. Individual cells have a moderate N:C ratio and generally contain a single oval nucleus (some bi- and trinucleated cells are also present). Nuclei are large, with smooth chromatin and 1–2 macronucleoli. Cytoplasm is moderate, lightly basophilic, rarely containing green/black round/rice grain-shaped granules (arrows). Low numbers of small lymphocytes and a few RBCs are present on a deeply basophilic background. These findings indicate a metastasis of a malignant neoplasm.

2 Based on the cytologic features of the metastatic cells, indicate the most likely differential diagnosis. Malignant melanoma (primary mucosal mass: confirmed as melanoma on histology section).

3 Which special stains could you use to confirm your diagnosis? Histochemical stains: Fontana–Masson Silver stain is often able to identify small amounts of melanin in largely amelanotic neoplasms). Immunohistochemical stains: Melan-A,

PNL2, TRP-1, and TRP-2 which are highly sensitive and specific for melanoma (sensitivity 100%, specificity 93.9%). S-100 is highly sensitive, but less specific because it may label a proportion of other neoplasia (soft tissue sarcomas).

4 Which tumors tend to metastasize to regional lymph nodes: carcinomas or sarcomas? Carcinomas tend to metastasize to lymph nodes; sarcomas typically metastasize via the hematogenous route rather than the lymphatic route.

Editors' note: The sensitivity and specificity of lymph node aspiration in the identification of metastases of solid tumors in dogs and cats may vary, depending on a number of factors. Sampling of a lymph node should include multiple aspirations and redirections in order to increase the probability of obtaining malignant cells when only a small focus of metastasis is present. In addition, in some cases, tumors may 'skip' lymph nodes along the channels of normal drainage and may not be present in those lymph nodes closest to the tumor. Some cases will present with lymph node enlargement as the primary sign and the identification of nonlymphoid malignancy within the lymph node is the first indication of an occult tumor. Some lymph nodes in the region of tumors may be enlarged and appear reactive on cytologic evaluation; the absence of malignant cells in these nodes cytologically or histologically does not rule out the possibility of more distant metastases.

In case of a malignant tumor, cytologic or histologic examination of regional lymph nodes should routinely be performed regardless of the size of those nodes. Previous studies on metastatic melanomas showed that up to 30% of lymph nodes with cytologic or histologic evidence of mandibular lymph node metastasis were normal in size and did not appear enlarged on clinical examination.

Further reading
Bankcroft JD, Stevens A (1996) (eds) *Theory and Practice of Histological Techniques*, 4th edn. Churchill Livingston, Edinburgh.
Gross TL, Ihrke PJ, Walder J (1992) (eds) *Veterinary Dermatohistopathology: A Macroscopic and Microscopic Evaluation of Canine and Feline Skin Disease*. Mosby, St. Louis, p. 464.
Lagenbach A, McManus PM, Hendrick MJ *et al.* (2001) Sensitivity and specificity of methods of assessing the regional lymph nodes for evidence of metastasis in dogs and cats with solid tumors. *Journal of the American Veterinary Medical Association* 218(9):1424–1428.

CASE 45

1 Which types of inflammatory cells can be seen in this BAL sample? The BAL sample contains a mixture of nondegenerate neutrophils and activated macrophages with abundant foamy cytoplasm, suggesting an active inflammatory response.

2 What are the structures indicated by the arrow in 45b? The slides contain frequent extracellular ovoid structures (cysts), which contain several small, basophilic bodies within them (trophozoites). Some of these organisms have been phagocytosed by macrophages. These can occur singly or in groups. These findings are consistent with *Pneumocystis carinii* infection. Cavalier King Charles Spaniel dogs with pneumocystis pneumonia have been documented to have significantly lower serum IgG concentrations and significantly higher serum IgM concentrations, suggesting a possible defect in immunity, which predisposes them to *Pneumocystis* infection.

Further reading
Watson PJ, Wotton P, Eastwood J *et al.* (2006) Immunoglobulin deficiency in Cavalier King Charles Spaniels with Pneumocystis pneumonia. *Journal of Veterinary Internal Medicine* 20:523–527.

CASE 46

1 Describe the features shown in the photomicrographs. There is a clear background with moderate numbers of RBCs and clear lipid vacuoles. Dense clusters of epithelial cells are observed, together with small numbers of neutrophils. The epithelial component shows features of malignancy which include: moderate anisokaryosis and anisocytosis, cellular crowding, and nuclear molding (conformity of adjacent cell nuclei to one another), with cellular dyscohesion (peripheral fragmentation). Very prominent, variably sized and also irregular, single to multiple nucleoli and coarsely stippled chromatin also are noted. There is deeply basophilic cytoplasm. All these findings support malignant proliferation. While there is active inflammation, the epithelial morphology is too pleomorphic to suggest only reactive hyperplasia or hypertrophy.

2 What is your interpretation of these findings? Pancreatic exocrine carcinoma. This is often metastatic, and screening for local nodal metastasis is strongly recommended. Compared with endocrine pancreatic pathology such as insulinoma, the exocrine epithelium has more basophilic, sometimes more purple to pink, grainy to granular cytoplasm, and can have tubular strands (not shown here), typically more pleomorphic with more malignant features.

CASE 47

1 What are these organisms? *Giardia* species cysts.
2 Describe how and where to look on the zinc sulfate fecal float to find the cysts. First check the entire slide for other parasite ova routinely at ×100. This gives

the *Giardia* cysts time to float to the top of the zinc sulfate solution. Increase magnification and scan carefully, just under the cover slip – air bubbles, especially small ones, are a useful landmark for finding the very top of the solution droplet beneath a cover slip. *Giardia* cysts, when they are numerous, will all be in the same plane of focus.

3 **Are yeast cells larger or smaller than these cysts? Do they float?** Yeast cells are very commonly mistaken for *Giardia* cysts, but are slightly smaller. Yeast will tend to sink to the bottom of the droplet.

CASE 48

1 **Describe the cytologic features seen in the FNA, and give an interpretation.** Clusters of well-differentiated hepatocytes are seen, most of which have indistinct cytoplasmic vacuolation. The cytoplasmic clearing caused by the vacuolation tends to be located in the periphery of the cell cytoplasm. These cytologic findings, together with the clinical history, are primarily suggestive of glycogen accumulation, likely due to steroid hepatopathy.

2 **Briefly discuss the biochemical profile. How does it support your cytologic findings?** Elevated ALT and AST are suggestive of mild hepatic damage. The markedly elevated ALP without an increase in bilirubin is typically drug induced, due to steroid hepatopathy. This can be due to exogenous corticosteroid administration or endogenous corticosteroid release, as seen in cases of Cushing's disease.

3 **Discuss additional diagnostic tests to confirm the underlying disease process.** A screening test such as the ACTH response test can be used to confirm a diagnosis of Cushing's disease. In this case the basal cortisol concentration was 221 nmol/l (ref. = 25–260 nmol/l) and the post-ACTH concentration was 745 nmol/l (ref. = 260–660 nmol/l). This is strongly suggestive of Cushing's disease. Dogs with iatrogenic Cushing's disease usually have both basal and post-ACTH cortisol concentrations of <221 nmol/l. An LDDS test can also be used. An HDDS test is needed to differentiate between pituitary-dependent hyperadrenocorticism and adrenal tumor. HDD suppresses more than 50% of pituitary tumors. If HDD does not suppress, measurement of endogenous ACTH levels is needed (<20 ng/ml is consistent with an adrenal tumor, >50 ng/ml is supportive of pituitary-dependent hyperadrenocorticism; 20–50 ng/ml is 'gray zone' or nondiagnostic). Ultrasound evaluation of the adrenals may also be helpful.

Editors' note: The interpretation of liver aspirate cytology is enhanced by knowledge of the clinical chemistry findings and endocrine testing, as illustrated in this case. Confidence in the interpretation of cytologic findings and elimination of various differential diagnoses is dependent on provision of pertinent case information. If the cytologic investigation is conducted before other studies, these features would indicate a need for additional investigation, and a chemistry profile and endocrine testing should be recommended.

Hepatocellular vacuolar change is also sometimes known as vacuolar hepatopathy or cytoplasmic rarefaction. It may be difficult to differentiate the 'fuzzy' vacuolation of glycogen accumulation and diffuse hydropic degeneration, while hepatic lipidosis is characterized by discrete, more crisply defined vacuoles. A PAS stain can be used to identify glycogen. Prior to diastase digestion, glycogen will stain bright pink with this stain. Following diastase digestion, glycogen will be removed and the pink staining reaction will be greatly decreased or absent.

CASE 49

1 Describe the cells present in the smear, and provide an overall interpretation. The samples are hypercellular. A significant percentage of cells present in the flecks is represented by round to oval plasma cells with a slight to moderate anisomacrocytosis, eccentrically placed, small, round nuclei, surrounded by moderate to large amounts of deeply basophilic cytoplasm, often showing a characteristic distinct paranuclear clear zone represented by the Golgi apparatus. In addition, some of these cells show irregular outline borders and a variable amount of distinct red color to the periphery of their cytoplasm, which is why they are referred to as 'flame cells'. Myeloid and erythroid precursors are present in low numbers, intermingled among the plasma cells. The presence of a high percentage of plasma cells is considered consistent with neoplasia.

2 What is your final interpretation, and what additional work up is needed to confirm the hypothesis? Multiple myeloma (MM). This is considered a myeloma-related disorder. The diagnosis of MM in dogs usually follows the demonstration of bone marrow plasmacytosis, the presence of osteolytic bone lesions (usually multiple bone marrow sites are involved), and the demonstration of serum or urine myeloma proteins (M component). All animals suspected of plasma cell tumors should receive a minimal diagnostic evaluation including a CBC, serum biochemistry profile, and urinalysis. If clinical hemorrhage is present, a coagulation assessment and serum viscosity measurements are indicated. Serum electrophoresis and immunoelectrophoresis are performed to determine the presence of a monoclonal component. A bone marrow core biopsy or multiple aspirations may be necessary due to the possibility of uneven clustering or infiltration of plasma cells in the bone marrow. Normal marrow contains less than 5% plasma cells, whereas myelomatous marrow often greatly exceeds this level. Current recommendations require more than 20% marrow plasma cells to be present. Skeletal radiographs are recommended to determine the presence and extent of osteolytic lesions, which may have diagnostic, prognostic, and therapeutic implications.

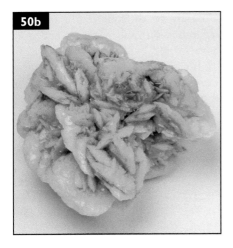

50b

CASE 50

1 What crystals are shown in the photomicrograph? The photomicrograph shows large numbers of calcium oxalate dihydrate (COD) crystals. Note the dipyramidal shape and the squares, whose corners are connected by perpendicular, refractile lines (envelope-like crystals). The image reveals marked crystal aggregation, which may be interpreted as a risk for urolith formation. In addition, numerous RBCs and few leukocytes can also be identified.

2 At what pH range do these crystals form? COD crystals form preferably at an acidic pH but can persist over a wide pH range and, therefore, may be present in alkaline urine. The factors promoting the formation of calcium oxalate uroliths are incompletely understood.

3 How can the hematuria be explained? The urolith was analysed by infrared spectroscopy and confirmed to be made of wheddelite (COD). These uroliths frequently have a rough surface with sharp protrusions (50b) and can damage the bladder's epithelium, resulting in hematuria.

CASE 51

1 Describe the features shown. There are a few columnar epithelial cells with a mat of intertwining fungal hyphae. The hyphae are narrow and septate.

2 What is your interpretation of these findings? These findings are consistent with a fungal infection of the equine uterus.

3 What is the significance of these findings? The diagnosis indicates that specific antifungal treatment is needed.

Candida species are frequently the cause of uterine fungal infections, but a number of opportunistic fungi may be involved in uterine infections.

Further reading
Freeman KP, Slusher SH, Roszel JF *et al.* (1986) Mycotic infections of the equine uterus. *Equine Practice* 8(1):34–42.
Roszel JF, Freeman KP (1988) Equine endometrial cytology. *Veterinary Clinics of North America: Equine Practice* 4:247–262.
Slusher SH, Freeman KP, Roszel JF (1985) Infertility diagnosis in mares using endometrial biopsy, culture and aspirate cytology. *Proceedings of the 31st Convention of the American Association of Equine Practitioners*, Toronto, p. 165.

CASE 52

1 Identify the organism. *Histoplasma capsulatum.*
2 What are the common routes of infection? Infection can occur by inhalation or ingestion of microconidia or macroconidia released from the mycelial form into the environment. Histoplasmosis is caused by the dimorphic fungus *Histoplasma capsulatum.* Cytologically, the organism is characterized by a 2–4 μm oval yeast organism with a thin clear halo (pseudocapsule). The organism has thin-based budding and is usually found within epithelioid macrophages. Budding forms are not commonly seen in cytologic preparations. Unlike *Coccidioides* and *Blastomyces*, *Histoplasma* is usually intracellular, within both macrophages and neutrophils. In addition, yeast-laden macrophages and neutrophils can be found on blood films with disseminated disease involving the bone marrow.

Further reading
Greene CE (2012) *Infectious Disease of the Dog and Cat*, 4th edn. Elsevier, St Louis, pp. 614–621.

CASE 53

1 Describe the main changes present in 53a? The large cell in the center of 53b represents a mononuclear phagocyte. Describe the organisms within the cytoplasm. What is your interpretation? There is a mixed population of lymphoid cells (small and intermediate/large forms), together with small numbers of mature plasma cells. Scattered macrophages are also noted. The cytoplasm of these cells contains 20–30 oval organisms approximately 3–5 μm in size with a red nucleus and pale blue cytoplasm representing amastigotes of *Leishmania infantum.* A red organelle, eccentric to the nucleus, is sometimes evident within the cytoplasm of these parasites. This is the kinetoplast, which is a distinctive feature of *Leishmania* organisms. This protozoal infection has a worldwide distribution and can cause different forms of disease in humans and animals (cutaneous, visceral, and mucocutaneous). Different species are transmitted by various species of *Phlebotomus*, the sandfly.

Answers

Leishmania infantum is endemic in Mediterranean countries. Dogs are the main reservoir of the parasite. Infection in cats has been documented but is rare. The promastigote is the parasitic stage in the sandfly, which infects the vertebrate host when bitten. Macrophages of the vertebrate host phagocytose the promastigotes, which starts intracellular replication as amastigotes. Macrophages die and release amastigotes, which enter other fixed or circulating macrophages. When a sandfly ingests blood containing infected macrophages from a vertebrate, amastigotes reproduce as promastigotes in the vector. Postinfection progression of the disease depends on host immune responses. Higher infectivity seems associated with lower proportions of T-helper cells. Many studies confirm the high incidence of asymptomatic infections in dogs living in endemic areas.

Direct observation of the parasite in lymph nodes, bone marrow, and skin aspirates/biopsy is the most reliable diagnostic test, but sensitivity is low (50–70%) and often no parasites can be detected. In these cases, cytology can be useful to exclude other diseases, such as lymphoma, which have a similar clinical presentation. There are ELISA and PCR tests for *Leishmania* that may be helpful in diagnosis of leishmaniasis.

2 Laboratory investigation revealed nonregenerative anemia, hyperglobulinemia characterized by polyclonal gammopathy, and mild renal azotemia. A coagulation panel was unremarkable. How can the epistaxis be explained? The endocellular parasite affects the mononuclear phagocyte system, often resulting in a strong immune system response and type III hypersensitivity (immune-complexes mediated), resulting in secondary renal, ocular, skin, and synovial damage. Laboratory investigation often reveals marked hyperglobulinemia and hypoalbuminemia, renal insufficiency, nephrotic syndrome, or glomerulonephritis. Serum protein electrophoresis is characterized by polyclonal gammopathy but monoclonal gammopathy has also been reported. Bleeding disorders are often observed in the course of canine leishmaniasis, particularly epistaxis. Epistaxis may be the only presenting sign, although thrombocytopenia is rarely observed. An acquired thrombocytopathy secondary to hyperglobulinaemia and hyperviscosity syndrome are hypothesized to be the underlying cause of this bleeding disorder.

CASE 54

1 Identify the structures indicated by the arrow. Acantholytic keratinocytes. The rounded epithelial cells with aqua-blue cytoplasm and small, round, reticulated nuclei and variable numbers of perinuclear vacuoles are consistent with acantholytic keratinocytes. Neutrophils are commonly associated with acantholytic keratinocytes in epithelial pustules. The acantholytic keratinocytes in the cytology correspond to these within the subcorneal pustule present in the histologic section (**54b**; H&E, ×40)

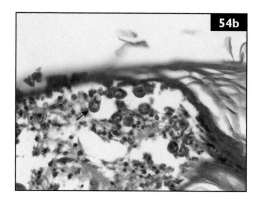

2 **List two differentials for this finding.** Pemphigus foliaceus, pemphigus erythematosus, and bullous impetigo can all present as pustular diseases with subcorneal pustules that contain acantholytic keratinocytes. In the case of impetigo, coccoid bacteria are often seen as well. Differentiation between pemphigus foliaceus and pemphigus erythematosus requires immunohistochemical stains that determine the distribution of immunoglobulins within the epithelium. Pemphigus foliaceus has intercellular localization of antibodies within the epidermis and pemphigus erythematosus has intercellular and basement membrane antibody localization.

Further reading
Gross LG, Ihrke PJ, Walder EJ *et al.* (2005) *Skin Diseases of the Dog and Cat: Clinical and Histopathologic Diagnosis*, 2nd edn. Wiley-Blackwell, Ames.

CASE 55

1 **Interpret the fluid specimen using the laboratory data and the photomicrograph.** Marked septic, mixed, mostly neutrophilic inflammation (peritonitis). The bacteria have been phagocytosed and are therefore significant. Free bacteria may or may not be contaminants.
2 **In view of the fact that the sample contained a pleomorphic bacterial population, including rods, cocci, and filamentous bacteria, select two further laboratory tests that you would like to run or be sent to a referral laboratory.** (1) Gram stain. These are gram-positive bacteria. Gram-negative (**1**) and gram-positive (**2**) bacteria, from two different lesions/patients, are shown in **55c** (Gram, ×100 oil). Gram staining allows the clinician to implement suitable interim antibiotics as part of a good therapeutic protocol. (2) Bacterial culture for both aerobes and anaerobes. A pleomorphic gram-positive bacterial population should alert the clinician to the possibility of *Actinomyces* or *Nocardia* infection.

119

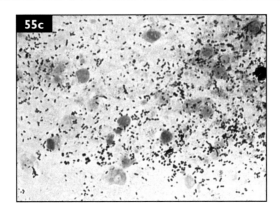

3 **What are the most common bacteria isolated from pyothorax and septic peritonitis?** Dogs: *Escherichia coli*, *Pasteurella* species, *Actinomyces* species. Cats: aerobes: *Pasteurella* species, *Actinomyces* species, *Escherichia coli*; anaerobes: *Bacteroides* species, *Peptostreptococcus anaerobius*, *Fusobacterium* species.

Editors' note: In some cases of pleural effusion due to *Actinomyces* or *Nocardia* infection, colonies of slender, beaded, filamentous or pleomorphic rods can be seen as soft, gray 'sulfur granules' with purulent exudate. These may be visible macroscopically, if large enough, as well as microscopically. Differentiation of *Nocardia* and *Actinomyces* is important, since different antibiotics are used for treatment. Standardization of Gram and acid-fast (Ziehl–Neelsen) staining techniques is important in obtaining consistent and reliable results.

Further reading
Walker AL, Jang SS, Hirsh DC (2000) Bacteria associated with pyothorax of dogs and cats: 98 cases (1989–1998). *Journal of the American Veterinary Medical Association* 216(3):359–363.

CASE 56
1 **What are the cells shown in the photomicrograph?** Moderately to markedly atypical columnar epithelial cells. Their nuclei are enlarged and have increased chromatin prominence. Small but distinct nucleoli are visible in several of the cells. Intercellular cohesion is observable, but cilia are not seen and normal orderly orientation and polarity of the cells are not preserved. Compare the features with those in **56b** (equine tracheal washing, Sano's modification of Pollack's Trichrome, ×50 oil). In this photomicrograph there is a cohesive group of columnar epithelial cells whose features are within normal limits.

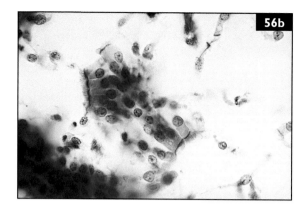

The nuclei are basal and uniform with delicate chromatin. Nucleoli are absent or inconspicuous. The terminal bar with attached cilia is easily seen at the luminal aspect of the columnar epithelial cells.

2 What is the significance of this finding? The epithelial atypia is significant since it indicates chronic, severe irritation to the airways. Without normal cells and cilia, the mucociliary apparatus and clearance mechanisms of the lung are compromised. In other fields there were numerous neutrophils. The features supported the clinical diagnosis of severe, chronic bronchopneumonia.

CASE 57

1 What is your cytologic interpretation? Mixed, purulent to pyogranulomatous inflammation with fungal hyphae.

2 List possible differentials for this organism. *Aspergillus*, *Penicillium*, *Chrysosporium*, and other hyalohyphomycetes. Determination of a specific species of fungus on cytologic and histologic preparations is difficult. The hyphae present in this specimen are septate, have acute angle branching, relatively uniform parallel sides, and occasional varices that resemble chlamydospores. The fungus in this case was identified by fungal culture of necropsy tissue (lung, abdominal mass, and abdominal lymph node) as *Aspergillus fumigatus*. The only diagnostic feature that can define a fungal agent as *Aspergillus* on cytology or histology is the presence of conidial heads. These structures are rarely found in tissues, but can be seen in tissue with high oxygen tension or within nasal turbinate tissue. Occasionally, small, blue–green to aqua staining conidia can be seen in aspirate cytology of *Aspergillus* lesions.

Editors' note: When commenting on possible identification of fungal elements in cytology, the species, breed, and clinical presentation, together with the morphology of the fungus, should be considered when providing a differential for the fungal species. However, fungal culture or molecular methods are needed for a definitive diagnosis.

Further reading
Lanzarin LD, Mariano LC, Macedo MC *et al.* (2015) Conidial heads (fruiting bodies) as a hallmark for histopathological diagnosis of angioinvasive aspergillosis. *Autopsy & Case Reports* 5:9–18.

CASE 58

1 What cell types are shown in the photomicrographs? The images show groups of large vacuolated epithelial cells, arranged in clusters, in a basophilic background containing RBCs. The cytoplasm is lightly basophilic with vacuolated cytoplasm. Nuclei are round, paracentral, and small, with dense chromatin. These findings are consistent with normal salivary gland tissue, which has been likely aspirated. Note that the mandibular lymph nodes are prone to accidental puncture due to their proximity to salivary glands.

2 Photomicrograph 58b shows a linear arrangement of the erythrocytes (indicated by the arrow), known as 'wind-rowing'. What is the cause of this? Wind-rowing is the result of a viscous background matrix. It can also be observed in other samples, including synovial fluid or FIP effusions, where the mucopolysaccharide or protein content, respectively, is expected to be high.

CASE 59

1 What is your interpretation based on cytologic observation? The cytologic findings are consistent with neutrophilic inflammation and intralesional *Cryptococcus neoformans* microorganisms.

2 What other diagnostic tests can be performed to support this diagnosis? Fungal culture can enable isolation and identification of the microorganisms if they are not found following cytologic examination of a case in which *Cryptococcus* infection is suspected, or if confirmation of a diagnosis is needed. Antigen detection using serum, urine, or CSF can be carried out to establish a diagnosis or for therapeutic monitoring: a titer as low as 1:1 is considered a positive test and diagnostic of cryptococcosis.

Cryptococcus infection and organisms may be seen in a variety of types of specimens, but in cats they are most commonly found in CSF or nasal specimens. They may be seen in cutaneous lesions or in pericardial, abdominal, or thoracic fluid, lymph node aspirates, respiratory cytology specimens, or other sites, depending on whether the infection is localized or generalized and the presenting signs and avenues of investigation.

Editors' note: *Cryptococcus* organisms may be confused with tissue cells since the central organism may resemble a nucleus and the surrounding halo or capsule may be mistaken for boundaries of cytoplasm. In some cases the organisms may be refractile and be confused with particles of glove powder, which may also be refractile. Sometimes, cryptococcal organisms are small and may not have a prominent capsule; these may be difficult to distinguish from lysed erythrocytes or air bubbles if present only in small numbers. The organisms may display a wide range of diameters (from 5 to 20 microns). Accompanying inflammation may vary from slight to absent or granulomatous. An apparent absence of inflammation cannot be relied on to rule out infection. Ultrastructurally, it has been shown that the capsule is formed by intertwined microfibrils radiating from the surface of the organism. A Mucicarmine or PAS stain will stain the surrounding capsule red or pink because of the mucopolysaccharide contents. The thickness of the capsule is believed to be related to the age and degree of degeneration of the organism, with younger, more well preserved elements showing less capsule. When budding is recognized, *Cryptococcus* will exhibit narrow-based budding.

CASE 60

1 Describe the cytologic findings, and give your cytologic interpretation. The smear contains several hepatocytes with round to oval nuclei and light basophilic cytoplasm. Large numbers of small lymphocytes are present around the hepatocytes and in the background. Lymphocytes are small round cells with a rim of basophilic cytoplasm. Nuclei are round and are about one to one and a half times the size of erythrocytes. Nuclear chromatin is dense and clumped. The cytologic findings are suggestive of a hepatic small cell lymphoma.

2 Discuss the condition. Many cats with hepatic lymphoma will present cytologically with high numbers of small lymphocytes. It is important to differentiate lymphocytic periportal hepatitis from hepatic lymphoma. Cats with hepatic lymphoma usually have severe hepatomegaly, whereas with lymphocytic periportal hepatitis, hepatomegaly is typically mild. Histologic confirmation is recommended in cats with severe lymphocytic infiltrates and marked hepatomegaly, regardless of the cytologic appearance of the lymphocytes. Hepatic infiltration due to chronic lymphocytic leukemia (CLL) will also have this appearance, so correlation with peripheral blood CBC and peripheral blood film morphology is needed. The distinction between CLL and small cell lymphoma with a leukemic phase may be difficult and may depend on evaluation of a number of body systems and organs.

Editors' note: It is important to include small cell lymphoma in your differential diagnosis list in addition to lymphocytic periportal hepatitis when lymphocytes are numerous in a liver aspirate.

CASE 61
Identify the exogenous and possible foreign body material in the photomicrograph (61; Wright–Giemsa, ×100 oil). The photomicrograph indicates paper fibers from a sticker fragment that resemble fungal hyphae but have no internal structures; they are more irregular and without branching.

CASE 62
1 Identify the main cell populations present in the smear, and describe the most relevant characteristics. In a clear background with frequent RBCs, there is a main population of small lymphoid cells. These have a small rim of basophilic cytoplasm, a round to indented nucleus, with granular chromatin and indistinct nucleoli. Immunophenotyping was performed and revealed a mixed population of T and B lymphoid cells, with a prevalence of T CD4+ cells, suggesting a non-neoplastic process. However, there are a few large nucleated cells (in the center of the photomicrograph) with abundant, irregularly microvacuolized cytoplasm and one or two round nuclei with reticular chromatin and small round nucleoli. These cells resemble human Reed–Sternberg cells of Hodgkin lymphoma. Reed–Sternberg cells generally stain negative to B-cell (CD20, CD79a) and T-cell (CD3, CD5) markers, but are supposed to derive from B-cell lineage in humans.
2 What is your interpretation? The cytologic aspects and the localization to a single cervical node are all suggestive of Hodgkin-like lymphoma. Differentials include reactive lymphoid hyperplasia and a histiocytic/dendritic cell disorder. However, the large binucleated cells are not expected with reactive lymphoid hyperplasia and are not classic for a histiocytic/dendritic cell disorder. Hodgkin lymphoma is a well recognized entity in humans and is rarely observed in domestic animals, mainly in the cat. In humans, differentials should include a T-cell-rich B-cell lymphoma (TCRBCL), a rare variant of large B-cell lymphoma, characterized by a prevalent population of non-neoplastic T cells with a B cell neoplastic expansion. In cats, differentiation of TCRBCL and Hodgkin-like lymphoma is challenging and specific criteria of differentiation have not been identified. Histology and immunohistochemistry are considered mandatory to confirm the cytologic suspicion of Hodgkin-like lymphoma in cats.

Further reading

Re D, Thomas RK, Behringer K *et al.* (2005) From Hodgkin disease to Hodgkin lymphoma: biologic insights and therapeutic potential. *Blood* **105**:4553–4560.

Walton RM (2001) Feline Hodgkin's-like lymphoma: 20 cases (1992–1999). *Veterinary Pathology* **38**:504–511.

CASE 63

1 What is the structure shown in the photomicrograph? An 'asbestos body'; the current preferred term is ferruginous body. These fibrillary structures have been associated with reaction to inhaled fibers of asbestos, but they may occur with inhalation of a number of different mineral fibers.

2 What is its significance? The significance of finding a ferruginous body in a tracheal washing from a horse is uncertain, since they are rarely observed. In humans they are linked to the development of mesotheliomas and bronchogenic carcinoma. Large numbers of ferruginous bodies in broncholavage fluid from humans probably reflect occupational exposure, whereas occasional bodies are a nonspecific finding. All inhabitants of modern urban societies have ferruginous bodies in their lungs, but usually the concentration in members of the general population is so low that they are rarely found in routinely prepared sections of lung or in respiratory cytology specimens. A Perl's Prussian Blue stain may increase sensitivity in detection of ferruginous bodies, since they often contain iron and stain positively (blue).

The finding of the ferruginous body in this horse may have been linked to his urban environment and working conditions. It is included in this book as an illustration of the variety of features that can be found when a large case volume is seen. Differential diagnoses may include other types of fibers from environmental contamination. These are not easily confused with plant material, since plant material usually contains visible cell walls.

In order to become familiar with the variety of contaminants that frequently occur with equine respiratory specimens (plant material, spores, pollen), collection of material by shaking of hay over a collection pot and leaving a slide sitting on a window ledge for several hours is recommended. The material collected in this manner can be prepared and stained for routine evaluation and provide examples of elements that commonly occur as environmental contaminants. The types of contaminants may vary between stables, ventilation systems, different batches of hay, management styles, and during various times of the year, so periodic evaluation of environmental contaminants is often useful for quality assurance and quality control with equine respiratory specimens.

CASE 64

1 Explain the abnormal RBC shape and the biochemistry abnormalities. Acanthocytes are spherical erythrocytes with blunt tipped spicules of different lengths projecting from the surface at irregular intervals. Abnormal amounts of lipid may accumulate in the outer half of the lipid bilayer during liver disease. This causes the membrane to evaginate and form spicules, resulting in acanthocytosis. The mild elevation in ALT and AST suggests minimal hepatic damage. Elevated bilirubin and ALP are indicative of cholestatic liver disease. Even mild elevations of serum ALP are significant in the cat because of the short half-life of the enzyme in this species.

2 Describe the cytologic findings, and give your cytologic interpretation. Several hepatocytes are seen, many of which contain distinct, punctate, clear cytoplasmic vacuoles. The nuclei of many of these hepatocytes are pushed to the periphery due to cytoplasmic vacuoles. Abundant punctate vacuoles are also noted in the background. The cytologic interpretation is vacuolar degeneration compatible with hepatic lipidosis.

3 List the differentials for your diagnosis. Hepatic lipidosis in cats may be a primary disease or may occur secondary to other metabolic, inflammatory, or neoplastic conditions. Approximately 50% of cases are reported to be idiopathic. Differentials for secondary hepatic lipidosis include diabetes mellitus, pancreatitis, hyperthyroidism, steroids, and neoplasia.

GGT measurement may help in the diagnostic process. A previous study showed that 80% of cats with lipidosis had increased ALP:GGT ratio.

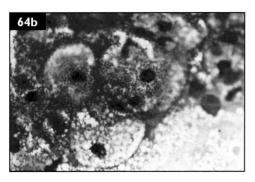

Editors' note: An additional photomicrograph is included here for comparison (64b; Wright–Giemsa, ×100 oil). The multiple small, crisply defined cytoplasmic vacuoles within hepatocytes are characteristic of this condition.

Further reading
Center SA, Baldwin BH, Dillingham S *et al.* (1986) Diagnostic value of serum gamma-glutamyl transferase and alkaline phosphatase activities in hepatobiliary disease in the cat. *Journal of the American Veterinary Medical Association* **188**(5):507–510.

CASE 65

1 Describe the cytologic findings, and give your cytologic interpretation. The smear contains hepatocytes with moderate to marked cytologic features of atypia including moderate anisocytosis, marked anisokaryosis, and single to multiple variably sized, round nucleoli. The chromatin pattern is clumped, with irregular margination. Binucleation and multinucleation are also present. These cytologic findings are suggestive of a hepatocellular neoplasia (e.g. hepatocellular carcinoma).

2 Discuss the various forms of this disease seen in the dog. Hepatocellular carcinoma is divided into diffuse, nodular, and massive forms. Grossly, the diffuse form consists of large areas of the liver infiltrated by nonencapsulated neoplastic tissue; the nodular form consists of multiple discrete nodules of variable size within several lobes; and a massive form consists of a large mass affecting a single liver lobe. Based on the ultrasound findings, the dog in this case likely had a diffuse form. Diffuse and nodular forms in the dog are associated with high metastatic potential (reported to be around 100% and 90%, respectively). The massive forms have relatively less metastatic potential (reported around 35%). Hepatocellular carcinomas usually maintain some degree of hepatocytic differentiation and can often be distinguished cytologically from metastatic hepatic neoplasms.

3 Discuss the prognosis for this patient. The prognosis for this patient is poor, based on the high potential for metastatic disease. Metastasis occurs most commonly to regional lymph nodes, peritoneum, and lungs. Hepatocellular carcinomas are also known to occasionally metastasize to the heart, spleen, kidney, intestine, brain, and ovary via the vascular system.

Editors' note: The diagnosis of hepatic neoplasia may be difficult, particularly in cases with moderate to severe liver disease. This may result in varying degrees of hepatocellular pleomorphism, which may result from degeneration, inflammation, and regeneration. A well-differentiated hepatocellular adenoma may resemble normal hepatocytes or have minimal atypia; histologic evaluation is usually required for a definitive diagnosis. A recent retrospective study on canine well-differentiated hepatocellular carcinomas identified a few characteristic cytologic features, which include: dissociation of hepatocytes, acinar or palisading arrangements of neoplastic cells, presence of naked nuclei and capillaries, together with mild anisocytosis, anisokaryosis, multinuclearity, and increased N:C ratios. If hepatic nuclei are stripped of cytoplasm, they may mimic metastatic or infiltrative neoplastic cells because of the presence of their characteristic prominent nucleolus, so care should be taken to evaluate cells with intact cytoplasm. Poorly differentiated hepatocellular carcinomas may be difficult to differentiate from metastatic carcinomas.

Further reading
Masserdotti C, Drigo M (2012) Retrospective study of cytologic features of well-differentiated hepatocellular carcinoma in dogs. *Veterinary Clinical Pathology* 41(3):382–390.

CASE 66

1 Describe the cell types and features illustrated in the two photomicrographs. There are a few erythrocytes and a low density of nucleated cells. The mucinous character of the background typical of synovial fluid is not apparent in these photomicrographs, but it was present when the glass slide was examined. In **66a** there are three small darkly stained cells that may be small lymphocytes or synoviocytes and two mononuclear cells with moderate amounts of basophilic cytoplasm containing clear intracytoplasmic vacuoles, which may be either synoviocytes or macrophages. **66b** shows a higher magnification, with two small dark cells that may be lymphocytes or small synoviocytes and a single reactive synoviocyte or macrophages with abundant foamy cytoplasm and clear intracytoplasmic vacuoles. No neutrophils or infectious agents are visible.

2 What is your interpretation of this case, and what are your comments? The fluid characteristics and the cytologic features are supportive of a nonsuppurative joint disease, likely degenerative joint disease (DJD). DJD is characterized by degeneration of the articular cartilage with secondary changes in associated joint structures. The disorder usually occurs secondary to osteochondrosis, joint instability, trauma, or joint dysplasia. A mild increase in the number of mononuclear cells in synovial fluid is the predominant finding.

Follow-up radiographs showed moderate osteoarthritic changes associated with both stifle joints. The alterations in synoviocytes may be quite subtle. Recognition of slight changes that may represent deviations from normal requires a careful study of synoviocytes found in normal joints. There is a limited range of changes that synoviocytes undergo in response to irritation or injury. Slight cytoplasmic enlargement, increased chromatin prominence, and slight nuclear enlargement are common and indicate increased activity. A variety of conditions may result in this appearance, but degenerative conditions should be included in the differential when this morphology is present. A good smear that is rapidly air dried, or a Papanicolaou-stained smear, is needed. If the smear is too thick and/or does not air dry rapidly, the cells may round up and stain darkly, and subtle changes may be difficult or impossible to appreciate.

CASE 67

1 What is the structure indicated by the arrow? There is an intranuclear rectangular crystalloid structure. Inclusions like this can be occasionally observed in liver aspirates from clinically healthy dogs and have an unknown clinical significance. However, these are felt to increase in association with chronic hepatic disorders.

Further reading
Maxie MG (2007) *Jubb, Kennedy, and Palmer's Pathology of Domestic Animals*, 5th edn. Saunders, Philadelphia, pp. 297–388.

CASE 68

1 What is the predominant cell type in photomicrograph 68a? The predominant cell type is osteoblasts. These cells can appear 'plasmacytoid' with eccentric nuclei and prominent perinuclear clear zones. Thus, even though this is a sarcoma, the neoplastic cells can be individualized and round in shape rather than occurring in groups with a spindloid shape characteristic of many other sarcomas. The nuclei here have fine chromatin and faint nucleoli can be observed.

2 What are the large multinucleated cells in photomicrograph 68b? The large multinucleated cells are osteoclasts, which can be associated with any lytic bone lesion. Additional osteoblastic cells are noted along with some more spindloid cells. In a different region of the smear, a loose aggregate of relatively uniform spindloid mesenchymal cells can be seen along with bright pink extracellular matrix (**68c**; Wright–Giemsa, ×20). Different histologic subtypes of osteosarcoma can have different cytologic appearances.

3 What is your most likely diagnosis? This cytology was most consistent with an osteoblastic osteosarcoma, which was confirmed by histopathology. Cytology has high correlation with histopathology for the detection of neoplasia in bone lesions, with higher cellular samples having higher concordance than low quality specimens.

4 What additional cytochemical stain could be performed to help assess the cell type of origin? Cytochemical staining for alkaline phosphatase (ALP) can help substantiate a bone origin (**68d**; ALP stain, ×20); however, it does not help distinguish between normal reactive and neoplastic bone tissue. ALP positivity

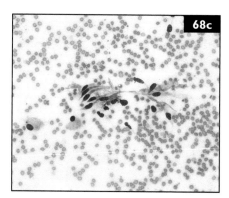

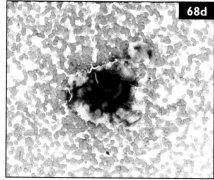

has also been observed in some other neoplastic tissues, including amelanotic melanoma, gastrointestinal stromal cell tumors, collision tumors, and anaplastic sarcomas.

Further reading

Berzina I, Sharkey LC, Matise I *et al.* (2008) Correlation between cytologic and histopathologic diagnoses of bone lesions in dogs: a study of the diagnostic accuracy of bone cytology. *Veterinary Clinical Pathology* 37:332–338.
Ryseff JK, Bohn AA (2012) Detection of alkaline phosphatase in canine cells previously stained with Wright-Giemsa and its utility in differentiating osteosarcoma from other mesenchymal tumors. *Veterinary Clinical Pathology* 41:391–395.

CASE 69

1 Describe the cytologic findings, and give your cytologic interpretation. The smear contains large numbers of hepatocytes, the majority appearing as bare nuclei embedded in a background of basophilic cytoplasm and crowded around a few intact hepatocytes; a microacinar pattern (indicated by the arrow) is also noted. These findings are suggestive of a well-differentiated hepatocellular carcinoma.

2 What additional tests might be useful in order to confirm the diagnosis? Surgical removal of the entire affected lobe and histologic examination led to a definitive diagnosis of fibrolamellar variant of well-differentiated hepatocellular carcinoma. Since evaluation of the tissue architecture and comparison with the normal liver parenchyma are needed for a histologic diagnosis of well-differentiated neoplasms, it is important to collect samples of adequate size, and possibly from the transition area immediately adjacent to the normal tissue. Diagnosis on small biopsy fragments can be very difficult or impossible.

Editors' note: Hepatocytes from well-differentiated hepatocellular carcinomas can be difficult to distinguish from normal/hyperplastic hepatocytes, and most of the time histopathology is required for a definitive diagnosis. However, specific cytologic features of well-differentiated hepatocellular carcinoma in dogs have been described and include dissociation of hepatocytes, acinar or palisading arrangements of neoplastic cells, and the presence of naked nuclei and capillaries, together with mild anisocytosis, anisokaryosis, multinucleation, and increased N:C ratio.

Further reading

Masserdotti C, Drigo M (2012) Retrospective study of cytologic features of well-differentiated hepatocellular carcinoma in dogs. *Veterinary Clinical Pathology* 41:382–390.

CASE 70

1 What type of fluid (fluid classification) is present in the abdomen? An exudate.
2 What are the cells shown in 70a? Neutrophils, reactive macrophages, and lymphocytes. Macrophages show signs of phagocytosis. Microorganisms are not seen.
3 What are the cells shown in 70b? The cell at the bottom center is a large lymphoid cell and many of the other cells have the appearance of poorly preserved lymphoid cells. A few of the cells in the center are neutrophils, occasionally showing intracytoplasmic coccoid microorganisms.
4 What is your interpretation? Mixed inflammation (peritonitis). This animal was found to have an encapsulated intra-abdominal abscess.

Editors' note: RIs for NCCs and classification of effusions in large animals differ from those for small animal specimens. (Guidelines for fluid classification in cows and horses are shown in Case 4.)

This case illustrates the importance of considering the proportions and absolute numbers of cell types and all the features in cytologic preparations. The finding of a few large lymphoid cells does not confirm the presence of malignancy, although it may raise the possibility of neoplasia.

The finding of many karyolytic neutrophils and intracellular bacterial cocci is consistent with an infectious and inflammatory condition. An intra-abdominal abscess should be considered when peritonitis is present. In some cases the abscess may be encapsulated and cause changes associated with irritation, while in others it may rupture or leak into the peritoneal cavity (as this case likely did) or contribute to generalized sepsis.

CASE 71

1 Review the laboratory data and photomicrograph, and give an appropriate interpretation. Lymphoma.
2 Given the young age of this cat and the anatomic location of the lymphoma, what other laboratory data would you like to obtain that may affect the prognosis of this patient? The cat's FeLV status. A large percentage of cats with thymic mediastinal lymphomas are FeLV positive. Cats with FeLV negative status have a better prognosis. This is currently under review as there is contradiction between early and current literature. Some publications claim that the discrepancy is related to the decreasing incidence of FeLV-related lymphoma due to vaccination and increased detection of antigenemic cats. This has shifted the demographics of lymphoma from affecting young FeLV-positive cats to more frequently affecting older FeLV-negative subjects.

Editors' note: The large discrete 'round cells' illustrated in this case are typical of neoplastic large lymphoid cells. Based on the age, presence of a mediastinal mass, and appearance of the cells, lymphoma is the correct interpretation.

Answers

Further reading
Duncan JR, Prasse KW, Mahaffey EA (1994) *Veterinary Laboratory Medicine: Clinical Pathology*, 3rd edn. Iowa State University Press, Ames, pp. 65–66.
Fabrizio F, Calam AE, Dobson JM *et al.* (2016) Feline mediastinal lymphoma: a retrospective study of signalment, retroviral status, response to chemotherapy and prognostic indicators. *Journal of Feline Medicine and Surgery* 16(8):637–644.
Hirschberger J, DeNicola DB, Hermanns W *et al.* (1999) Sensitivity and specificity of cytologic evaluation in the diagnosis of neoplasia in body fluids from dogs and cats. *Veterinary Clinical Pathology* 28(4):142–146.

CASE 72

1 What can be seen in the smear? Refractile crystalline material of various sizes. In other fields (not illustrated) there are a few spindle cells and macrophages. A few multinucleated macrophages are also present.

2 What is your interpretation? Calcinosis circumscripta (also called calcium gout, apocrine cystic calcinosis, or tumoral calcinosis). This condition is considered to be a subcategory of calcinosis cutis. Its etiopathogenesis is poorly understood. It occurs primarily in young, large-breed dogs and a predisposition in German Shepherd Dogs has been identified. It has been reported in the cervical spine, with spinal cord compression, the tongue, and the skin, particularly on the extremities, adjacent to joints, and over pressure points. Boxers and Boston Terriers may be predisposed to lesions at the base of the pinna and on the cheek.

The lesions are usually single but some cases have multiple or bilaterally symmetrical lesions. The amount of crystalline material and associated granulomatous and fibroblastic response may vary amongst individuals; however, abundant crystalline material is usually present, as shown in this case. The radiographic and histologic appearances are also characteristic. Treatment involves surgical removal and lesions have not been reported to recur following surgery.

In humans, calcinosis circumscripta has been associated with hyperphosphatemic imbalance and is considered to be familial. It has not been determined whether such an imbalance may play a role in some cases of calcinosis circumscripta in dogs.

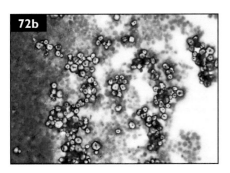

The irregular crystalline material obtained from aspirates of foci of calcinosis circumscripta must not be confused with the starch crystals that are contaminants from powdered gloves (**72b, c**; Wright–Giemsa, ×25 oil and ×100 oil, respectively). Starch crystals are small and oval to angular. At high magnification a characteristic central cross, slit, or oval structure can be seen. Glove powder is a frequent contaminant of cytologic specimens collected when gloves are worn or in an area where powdered gloves are used. When found in a body cavity fluid specimen with granulomatous inflammation or history of a mass, the possibility of a talc-associated granuloma from previous contamination with glove powder should be considered.

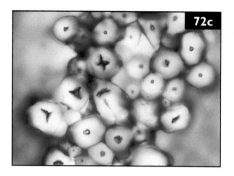

CASE 73

1 Identify the organism. *Coccidioides* species (either *C. immitis* or *C. posadasii*).
2 Identify the structures labeled 1 and 2. Spherule (1); endospore(s) (2).
3 What are the two most common organ systems affected by this disease in the dog? The respiratory and musculoskeletal systems are the most commonly affected organ systems in the dog.

Coccidioidomycosis is a deep fungal disease caused by the morphologically identical but genetically unique dimorphic fungi *C. immitis* and *C. posadosii*. The primary route of infection is inhalation, with rare cases of transdermal inoculation. In cytologic preparations, the organism is characterized by a basophilic spherule with a thick cell wall that often has a folded appearance and, in larger spherules, shows endosporulation. The spherules can be up to 120 microns in diameter. The organism is typically associated with purulent to pyogranulomatous inflammation.

Further reading
Nguyen C, Barker BM, Hoover S *et al.* (2013) Recent advances in our understanding of the environmental, epidemiological, immunological, and clinical dimensions of coccidioidomycosis. *Clinical Microbiology Reviews* 26:505–525.
Shubitz LF (2007) Comparative aspects of coccidioidomycosis in animals and humans. *Annals of the New York Academy of Sciences* 1111:395–403.

CASE 74

1 Based on these photomicrographs, describe the cells. Are they consistent with normal renal tissue? This densely cellular sample consists of many extremely large, round to oval cells characterized by scant to moderate pale basophilic cytoplasm that often contains variable numbers of fine clear vacuoles. Note the size of the cells compared with background neutrophils. Most cells contain a single round to oval to irregular nucleus, paracentrally located; however, scatted multinucleated cells are also observed. Anisocytosis and anisokaryosis are moderate to marked. An atypical mitotic figure is also noted (**74b**). In the submitted sample there is no evidence of renal tissue.

2 What is the most likely cytologic diagnosis? The most likely cytologic diagnosis based on cellular morphology and tissue distribution is an histiocytic sarcoma, which appears to be disseminated, based on the clinical presentation. The typical cytologic features of histiocytic sarcoma include sheets of large, pleomorphic round cells with prominent multinucleated cells, marked cytologic atypia, and bizarre mitotic figures. Cytophagia may be observed in some variants.

3 What tests could be performed to confirm this diagnosis? Additional tests are recommended for definitive diagnosis and include histopathology. The latter was performed and confirmed the cytologic diagnosis. Special immunohistochemical stains can also be helpful to further corroborate the cytologic and histologic diagnosis. The biopsies from this dog were strongly positive for CD204, a histiocytic marker. Neoplastic cells in histiocytic sarcoma are also positive for other markers, including CD1a, CD11c, MHCII, and CD18.

Articular histiocytic sarcoma can present as a localized disease potentially cured by surgical excision early in disease progression; however, widespread involvement is eventually possible, as was observed in this dog. Hemophagocytic variants can be characterized by regenerative anemia and thrombocytopenia, which were not present. This presentation can be misinterpreted as Evan's syndrome. The clients elected palliative care for this dog based on the widespread disease.

Further reading
Moore PF (2014) A review of histiocytic diseases of dogs and cats. *Veterinary Pathology* 51:167–184.

CASE 75

1 Describe the cell population in the photomicrograph. In a clear background with frequent RBCs, a single population of large pleomorphic lymphoid cells can be observed. These show abundant, lightly basophilic cytoplasm containing multiple purple to magenta granules of different sizes. Nuclei are large (>2.5 times the diameter of RBCs), round to oval, occasionally indented, with granular chromatin and small poorly visible nucleoli.

2 What is your interpretation? Large granular lymphocyte (LGL) lymphoma. LGL lymphoma is a high-grade subtype of lymphoma in the cat, often involving the gastrointestinal tract and/or mesenteric lymph nodes. Cells have a T-cell phenotype, in addition to the presence of the intracytoplasmic granules, and are positive to CD3, CD5, often CD8 alpha-alpha, and rarely CD4. Eosinophils may occasionally be observed, intermingled with neoplastic LGL. LGL lymphoma has an aggressive clinical behavior in the cat; blood and/or bone marrow involvement is a common finding at the time of the diagnosis.

Further reading
Roccabianca P, Vernau W, Caniatti M *et al.* (2006) Feline large granular lymphocyte (LGL) lymphoma with secondary leukemia: primary intestinal origin with predominance of a CD3/CD8(alpha)(alpha) phenotype. *Veterinary Pathology* 43:15–28.

CASE 76

1 What cells are present? The smear contains a monomorphic population of large lymphoid cells. These have small amounts of lightly basophilic granular cytoplasm and a round, paracentral nucleus, occasionally indented, with coarse granular chromatin and multiple small round nucleoli.

2 What is your interpretation? Large cell lymphoma.

CASE 77

1 What are the structures shown in the smears? Calcium carbonate and calcium oxalate dihydrate crystals. The calcium carbonate crystals are the rounded structures. Radiating striations from the central core are visible in many crystals in the higher-magnification figure. The rectangular/square crystals with a central cross (like an envelope) are the calcium oxalate dihydrate crystals.

2 What is the significance of these findings? The calcium carbonate crystals are within normal limits in equine urine. Horses absorb calcium from the intestinal tract and eliminate excess calcium in the urine. The calcium oxalate dihydrate crystals may also be within normal limits and tend to appear when the animal is eating oxalate-containing plants.

3 What is your interpretation? The interpretation of this specimen is: no abnormality detected. The findings are within normal limits. In some cases excessive irritation may be associated with marked crystalluria, but other possible causes for urinary tract-related clinical signs, such as urolithiasis, should be ruled out. Furthermore, polyuria and polydipsia may be very difficult to document in the horse due to variation in water drinking associated with environmental conditions, exercise, diet, and exercise.

Answers

CASE 78

1 **What are your differential diagnoses?** The viscous appearance and alignment of RBCs evident at low power suggest a mucinous matrix associated with this neoplasm. The spindle shape of the cells and numerous nuclear features of atypia suggest a malignant mesenchymal tumor, most likely a myxosarcoma. Nuclear criteria of malignancy include: anisokaryosis, occasional multinucleation (78a, center), variable N:C ratio, nuclear fragmentation, prominent nucleoli, and chromatin smudging. Alcian Blue staining of the ground substance for mucin may help to confirm the diagnosis. Several other tumors can be characterized by a myxomatous matrix and could be included in a differential diagnosis (e.g. chondrosarcoma, chordoma, or myxoid liposarcoma). These tumors can usually be differentiated by their cytologic and histologic features.

CASE 79

1 **Describe the cytologic findings and give your cytologic interpretation.** There are a few isolated very large cells and a small cluster of similar cohesive cells organized in a pavimentous pattern, together with frequent small lymphocytes. These large cells have a lightly blue cytoplasm, with angular borders, and round central nuclei with granular chromatin. Anisocytosis is marked. Observation of large cohesive epithelial cells in a lymph node aspirate is highly suggestive of metastatic carcinoma. The abundant cytoplasm with defined angular borders is supportive of a squamous origin.

Preoperative cytologic evaluation of FNAs of regional lymph nodes is useful for neoplastic staging and highly correlates with the histologic results.

Further reading
Herring ES, Smith MM, Robertson JL (2002) Lymph node staging of oral and maxillofacial neoplasms in 31 dogs and cats. *Journal of Veterinary Dentistry* **19**:122–126.

CASE 80

1 **The cells seen in the photomicrographs are most consistent with what general cell lineage?** The loose aggregates of cells, which are oval to spindloid with indistinct cell margins, are most consistent with a mesenchymal origin.

2 **Given the tissue distribution of the lesions, the clinical history, and the hematologic data, what is the most likely specific neoplasm in this dog?** The cytologic features, together with the clinical history, the evidence of regenerative anemia, and mild thrombocytopenia are considered suspicious for hemangiosarcoma. Cytology alone cannot reliable distinguish hemangiosarcoma from other soft tissue sarcomas; however, intratumoral or intracavitary bleeding can characterize

intermittent rupture of these lesions, which are formed by abnormal neoplastic vascular structures. Although not specific for hemangiosarcoma, the presence of hemosiderin-laden macrophages within lesions (80c; Wright–Giemsa, ×100 oil) is often considered characteristic because of the tendency for bleeding. Neoplastic cells in hemangiosarcoma can also show signs of erythrophagocytosis. Erythrophagocytosis has also been reported in other mesenchymal neoplasms, including hemophagocytic histiocytic sarcoma and osteosarcoma.

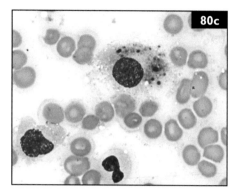

Because of the disseminated nature of the lesions, surgery was not considered an option, and the patient was treated with palliative chemotherapy.

Further reading
Barger AM, Skowronski MC, MacNeill AL (2012) Cytologic identification of erythrophagocytic neoplasms in dogs. *Veterinary Clinical Pathology* 41:587–589.

CASE 81
1 Is this a parasite? No. It is a fairly common pseudoparasite in dog feces.
2 What is it? A yeast, *Cyniclomyces guttulatus* (*Saccharomycopsis guttulatus*). Owners report that many dogs that pass this organism eat rabbit feces.

CASE 82
1 Identify the structures/cells labeled 1, 2, 3, and 4, and state their significance. 1 = erythrophagocytosis (can occur in transit with unfixed fluid specimens or *in vivo*); 2 = hemosiderin (is a more stable but less available form of iron, composed of ferritin and denatured ferritin protein in lysosomes); 3 = bilirubin crystals (these are the primary end product of heme degradation in most mammals, by the conversion of biliverdin to bilirubin by biliverdin reductase); 4 = hematoidin crystals (these are an insoluble crystalline form of bilirubin, chemically identical to bilirubin). Sometimes referred to as 'tissue bilirubin', hematoidin forms when oxygen tension is low (hypoxic conditions). Heme oxygenase, the enzyme that cleaves the tetrapyrrole heme ring once the amino acids and iron are liberated, uses molecular oxygen and NADPH. Therefore, hematoidin is often observed with tissue or intracavity hemorrhage in mammals (see **82d** for a flow diagram of RBC breakdown within a macrophage).

137

Answers

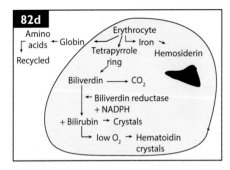

82d

Amino acids → Globin
Recycled

Erythrocyte
↓ ↓ → Iron →
Tetrapyrrole   Hemosiderin
ring

Biliverdin ——→ CO_2

← Biliverdin reductase
  + NADPH
+ Bilirubin → Crystals

↳ low O_2 → Hematoidin
              crystals

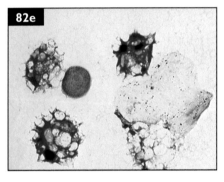

82e

2 Which of the findings indicate chronic hemorrhage? 2, 3, and 4. Not 1, because it can occur in transit unless the specimen is fixed with formalin or 40% ethanol immediately following collection. Papanicolaou or H&E staining are required for fixed specimens and may not be available from all laboratories.

3 Which special stain would you request to confirm that hemosiderin (labeled 2) from blood breakdown pigment is present and contains iron? Perl's Prussian Blue stain: stains iron blue to black (82e; Perl's Prussian Blue, ×100 oil). The blue to blue–black staining within macrophages indicates the presence of iron.

4 List three common causes of hemorrhagic effusions and relevant laboratory tests you can use in the investigation of causes of hemorrhagic effusions. Considerations for hemorrhagic effusions should include: coagulopathy (check platelets and test APTT and PT from clotting cascade); trauma (clinical history and external signs); or neoplasia (diagnostic imaging and identification of possible internal or external masses or other abnormalities warranting further investigation).

Editors' note: Other differential diagnoses that should be considered with hemorrhagic effusions include vascular rupture or compromise, organ torsion, rodenticide toxicity, or iatrogenic contamination. In some cases, iatrogenic contamination may be easily differentiated from true hemorrhage, but in others it may be difficult or impossible to differentiate unless features supporting hemorrhage, such as presented in this case, are present. Iatrogenic contamination is supported by a change from clear or yellow to bloody as the specimen is aspirated. The presence of platelets in the smears supports iatrogenic contamination or very recent hemorrhage, since they disappear rapidly from fluids containing blood. In fluids containing true hemorrhage the sample seldom clots and platelets are rarely seen unless very recent hemorrhage (within the last several hours) has occurred. In fluid specimens immediately fixed in 40–50% ethanol or with 10%

formalin for Papanicolaou-stained preparations immediately after collection, the presence of erythrophagocytosis supports recent hemorrhage since fixation prevents phagocytosis of erythrocytes during specimen transport.

Further reading
Meyer DJ, Harvey JW (1999) *Veterinary Laboratory Medicine: Interpretation and Diagnosis*, 2nd edn. WB Saunders, Philadelphia, p. 260.

CASE 83

1 Describe the cytologic findings. There is a slight protein background with several crystals that are flat, clear plates with 'notched corners'. These are consistent with cholesterol crystals.
2 What is the significance of these findings? Cholesterol crystals may be seen in cysts with static secretion. They may be seen in areas with increased cell turnover and breakdown of lipid-containing cell membranes.
3 What is your cytologic interpretation, and what are your comments? Based on the cytologic features, the interpretation would be consistent with origin from a secretory cyst. There is no current indication of inflammation or infection. Cells that would suggest a lining for, or origin for, a cyst are not seen. The possibility of an adjacent tumor that is not represented in this collection cannot be ruled out, but many cysts with this cytologic appearance are non-neoplastic in origin. They are not expected to resolve spontaneously; therefore, surgical removal with histologic evaluation should be considered.

CASE 84

1 What is the very large cell present in 84a? A mature megakaryocyte. These very large cells are platelet precursors and are characterized by having abundant blue cytoplasm with poorly defined borders and multiple fused round nuclei.
2 What are the small cells indicated by the arrows in 84b? The cells indicated by the arrows are mature plasma cells. They appear as round cells, with moderate amounts of deeply blue cytoplasm, a clear perinuclear area (Golgi zone), and defined cytoplasmic borders. They also have an eccentric nucleus with a condensed chromatin pattern and poorly distinct nucleoli. In the bone marrow sample from this dog, plasma cells were 10% of all nucleated cells (<2% in normal bone marrow samples), indicating the presence of plasma cell hyperplasia.
3 What diseases can cause an increase in these cells in the bone marrow? Plasma cell hyperplasia may occur secondary to chronic inflammatory conditions, including canine ehrlichiosis. This benign proliferation must be differentiated from multiple myeloma, which is a neoplastic proliferation of plasma cells within the

bone marrow, often accompanied by monoclonal gammopathy, radiologic evidence of bone lysis, and Bence Jones proteinuria. In multiple myeloma, the plasma cell proportion in bone marrow is >15%, with plasma cells frequently occurring in sheets, sometimes with atypical morphology. This dog had a positive IgG titer for *Ehrlichia canis*, and was treated with doxycycline.

Further reading
Kuehn NF, Gaunt SD (1985) Clinical and hematologic findings in canine ehrlichiosis. *Journal of the American Veterinary Medical Association* **186**:355–358.

CASE 85

1 Describe the cytologic findings observed in photomicrograph 85a. There is a clear background with few to moderate extracellular metachromatic (magenta) granules and occasional RBCs. A small group of well-granulated mast cells is noted. Mast cells have moderate amounts of cytoplasm, with distinct borders, filled with metachromatic granules that partially obscure the nuclei. These, when visible, are round and centrally to paracentrally located. Nuclear details cannot be appreciated. One eosinophil is observed in the lower left quadrant.

2 What is your interpretation? Mast cell tumor (MCT).

3 Name the cell labeled 1 and describe the structure labeled 2 in photomicrograph 85b. Reactive mesenchymal cell (fibroblast) (1), indicative of fibroplasia. The structure labeled 2 indicates hyalinized collagen bundles, consistent with degraded collagen or collagenolysis.

The presence of eosinophils, degraded collagen, and fibroplasia are all common findings in MCTs, and are secondary to the release of histamine, proteolytic enzymes, and chemokines from the granules of the mast cells.

Editors' note: Clinical staging is recommended after a diagnosis of MCT has been reached. This includes a CBC (to identify possible systemic mastocytosis), cytologic assessment of regional lymph nodes, and abdominal ultrasound (with cytologic evaluation of spleen and liver if abnormalities are detected). A cytologic grading scheme has been recently published. MCTs are considered high grade if poor granulation is identified or if there are two of the following cytologic features: presence of any mitotic figures, anisokaryosis >50%, bi/multinucleation, or nuclear pleomorphism. This proposed cytologic grading scheme has been found to be predictive of survival and correlates with the 2-tier histologic grading system.

Wide surgical excision with histopathologic examination is the main treatment option; cryosurgery, radiotherapy, and/or chemotherapy may also be considered. Prognostic factors for MCTs in dogs include clinical stage, histologic grade, proliferation markers (e.g. Ki67, AgNORs), and the presence of a c-Kit mutation.

Further reading
Blackwood L, Murphy S, Buracco P *et al.* (2014) European consensus document on mast cell tumours in dogs and cats. *Veterinary Comparative Oncology* **10**:1–29.
Camus MS, Priest HL, Koehler JW *et al.* (2016) Cytologic criteria for mast cell tumour grading in dogs with evaluation of clinical outcome. *Veterinary Pathology* pii. 03009858 16638721 [E-pub ahead of print]

CASE 86

1 What are your differential diagnoses? Allergic and parasitic bronchitis/ bronchopneumonitis are the two most likely diagnoses.

2 What other diagnostic test(s) do you recommend? Careful examination of multiple slides for parasitic larvae is indicated. If none are found, a fecal Baermann's flotation test should be performed as the parasite may be swallowed when the dog coughs up sputum. Bronchoscopic examination may reveal the presence of parasitic nodules at the bifurcation of the trachea with *O. osleri* infection. These may also be observed on radiographs. Allergic bronchitis is diagnosed by exclusion of parasitic infection and a response to corticosteroid therapy, as well as identification of an allergen, if possible, in the animal's environment.

Editors' note: Other less common differential considerations should include the possibility of pulmonary eosinophilic infiltrates, which may be focal. These may be idiopathic or associated with heartworm disease. Some types of tumor (mast cell tumor, T-cell lymphomas, or some types of epithelial and mesothelial malignancies) have also been associated with eosinophilic infiltrates, but would be differentiated by localizing clinical signs and histories that vary from that given in this case. It may be very difficult to determine an inciting antigen in cases of allergy to inhaled antigens.

CASE 87

1 Describe what you see in these smears. There are groups of epithelial cells with oval, hypochromatic 'bland' nuclei without granular chromatin or nucleoli. The cytoplasm is insubstantial and the boundaries are indistinct. The nuclei are often overlapping or very close together.

2 What is your interpretation of these findings? These features are consistent with inactivity of winter anestrus.

3 Why is this good to know? This is good to know because it indicates that this mare is not ready to breed. The mare may need to be put under light or undergo hormone treatment, or it may be necessary to wait for her to come naturally into active reproductive physiologic activity.

Answers

CASE 88

1 Describe the features shown in the photomicrographs, and provide a general description. Samples are highly cellular with adequate preservation. The background is clear and contains moderate numbers of RBCs. There are a few cohesive clusters of hepatocytes arranged in regular sheets (1). These cells have abundant, granular basophilic cytoplasm, rarely containing clear punctate vacuoles, and greenish–brown intracytoplasmic granules. A few dark ribbons of inspissated bile, which form casts within the biliary canaliculi, are also noted (2). In addition, there are also variable numbers of hematopoietic cells, mostly erythroid, at different stages of maturation. The erythroid cell line is characterized by rubriblasts (3) (large round cells with moderate amounts of deeply basophilic cytoplasm and a round, paracentral nucleus, with coarse granular chromatin) and rubricytes and metarubricytes (4) (small cells, part of the maturative compartment, characterized by small amounts of basophilic cytoplasm and small hyperchromatic and pyknotic nuclei). These cells are often present in small cohesive clusters, associated with macrophages (hematopoietic islands). Rare large multinucleated cells (megakaryocytes, from which platelets are derived) (5) also are noted.

2 What is your final interpretation? Hepatic extramedullary hematopoiesis. Evidence of hepatic hematopoiesis can be observed in dogs with ongoing anemia or in nonanemic dogs with chronic hepatitis. This may be part of a nonspecific reaction, likely due to local tissue changes that create a hospital microenvironment that allows growth and differentiation of hematopoietic stem cells. Occasionally, similar findings may also be observed in nodular regenerative hyperplasia. Moreover, the presence of a liver mass containing a mixture of hematopoietic precursor cells, together with well-differentiated adipocytes, may suggest a myelolipoma, which is an infrequent canine hepatic neoplasm.

CASE 89

1 What cell types can be identified in the photomicrograph, and how would you describe this cell arrangement? There are occasional erythrocytes and moderate numbers of large mononuclear cells, most likely synoviocytes, in a pink granular background. Those cells show a linear arrangement, referred to as wind-rowing, frequently observed in high viscosity samples such as synovial fluid or salivary gland aspirates.

2 What is your diagnosis? The cytologic interpretation is consistent with degenerative joint disease.

Degenerative joint disease (osteoarthritis, osteoarthropathy) is characterized by degeneration of joint structures secondary to conditions such us joint instability due to ligament injury or developmental diseases. Changes in the synovial fluid may include decreased viscosity and protein concentration and normal to poor mucin clot formation. Cellularity is often increased (up to 10×10^9/l) with a predominance of mononuclear cells (>90%), typically macrophages or enlarged synovial lining cells, found isolated or in thick sheets. Small numbers of lymphocytes and rare nondegenerate neutrophils may be seen. The concurrent presence of osteoclasts may suggest erosion of the cartilage and/or bone.

Editors' note: The slightly atypical sinovial lining cells seen in this case are sometimes referred to as hyperplastic and hypertrophic sinovial lining cells, because they are enlarged compared with small synoviocytes and have increased chromatin prominence and foci of increased layers of synoviocytes histologically.

This cytologic finding is not specific for osteoarthritis but is consistent with a response to ongoing irritation. A clinical diagnosis of degenerative joint disease/ osteoarthritis requires correlation with other findings, such as clinical history, radiography, and response to various treatments.

CASE 90
1 What are the main differentials with this pulmonary pattern, cytologic findings, and peripheral eosinophilia? Differential diagnoses for a dog with diffuse interstitial pulmonary pattern and peripheral eosinophilia include migration of intestinal parasites, lungworm infection, hypereosinophilic syndrome, and allergic pneumonitis.

The lungworm observed here is *Aleurostronglylus abstrusus*. It is common in cats and the intermediate hosts are snails and slugs. The disease process is often self-limiting, although some cats do require therapy. This cat was an indoor-outdoor cat that had been missing for 1 week, 8 weeks prior to developing the cough. The prepatent period for *A. abstrusus* infection is 6–18 weeks.

CASE 91
1 Describe the cells and features seen in the smear. There are many cohesive papillary groups and rafts of cells. Some acinar configurations, with cells arranged around a clear space that is likely to be a lumen, are apparent. These cells have oval nuclei, usually with single small but distinct nucleoli. The cytoplasm is scant to moderate and varies from homogeneous to vacuolated. Some cells contain a single large cytoplasmic vacuole, while others contain multiple small vacuoles.
2 What is your interpretation of this aspirate? The cytologic features are consistent with an epithelial lesion of mammary origin. A mammary neoplasm is a primary consideration, although histologic confirmation is recommended. Cytology lacks adequate sensitivity and specificity for the diagnosis of mammary neoplasms, especially when cytologic features of malignancy are not very marked.

Answers

Histopathology is recommended in these cases for further characterization. A mammary adenocarcinoma was confirmed on histopathology.

Mammary adenocarcinomas are uncommon neoplasms in the mare. Often, many neutrophils are present (not seen in this case) because there is concurrent mastitis; therefore, it may be difficult to diagnose in cases with overwhelming inflammation and few cells with features of malignancy. In this case a large number of malignant cells were obtained and confidence in the cytologic diagnosis of mammary malignancy was high.

Further reading
Freeman KP (1993) Cytologic evaluation of the equine mammary gland. Satellite article. *Equine Veterinary Education* 5(4):212–213.

Freeman KP, Slusher SH, Roszel JF *et al.* (1988) Cytologic features of equine mammary secretions: normal and abnormal. *Compendium on Continuing Education for the Practicing Veterinarian* 10(9):1090–1100.

CASE 92
1 Describe the cells represented in the photomicrographs. In a clear background with moderate numbers of RBCs and a few lymphoglandular bodies, there is a main population of medium and large lymphoid cells (1). These cells are medium to large (nuclei ≥2 times the diameter of RBCs), with moderate amounts of clear blue cytoplasm, often visible perinuclear halo, and rarely forming small cytoplasmic tails. Nuclei are pleomorphic, mostly round, occasionally indented, or paracentral to eccentric, with irregularly clumped fine chromatin. Nucleoli are inconspicuous and only rarely visible. Rare small lymphocytes (2) are scattered amongst the neoplastic cells, and a mature plasma cell (3) is recognized in the center of the picture. Frequent atypical mitotic figures are also noted (4).

2 What is your interpretation? High-grade lymphoma.

3 Which is the likely immunophenotype? The cytologic features are overall suggestive of a high-grade T-cell lymphoma. Immunophenotyping remains mandatory to define subtype and predict prognosis; however, cell lineage may be suspected based on cytology. The cellular pleomorphism, together with the presence of elongated cytoplasm, indented to convoluted nucleus, and poorly identifiable nucleolus, suggest a T-cell phenotype. Flow cytometric (or immunohistochemical) analysis on cases like this commonly shows positivity to T-cell markers (CD3, CD5, CD4 or, more rarely, CD8) and none to B-cell markers. According to the updated Kiel classification this lymphoma is classified as pleomorphic large cell lymphoma, and peripheral T-cell lymphoma on histology. This lymphoma subtype is usually clinically highly aggressive, with variable median survival times, generally not exceeding 7–8 months, and a limited response to chemotherapy in comparison with

B-cell forms. Hypercalcemia may be associated with high-grade T-cell lymphoma and, more rarely, paraneoplastic eosinophilia may also be observed.

Further reading
Ponce F, Marchal T, Magnol JP *et al.* (2010) A morphological study of 608 cases of canine malignant lymphoma in France with a focus on comparative similarities between canine and human lymphoma morphology. *Veterinary Pathology* **47**:414–433.
Rebhun RB, Kent MS, Borrofka SA *et al.* (2011) CHOP chemotherapy for the treatment of canine multicentric T-cell lymphoma. *Veterinary Comparative Oncology* **9**:38–44.

CASE 93

1 Describe the findings seen in the photomicrograph. The aspirate harvested a monomorphic population of round discrete cells in a clear background, with occasional RBCs. These cells have moderate amounts of lightly basophilic cytoplasm; nuclei are round, central to paracentrally located, with a finely stippled chromatin pattern. Nucleoli are absent or poorly visible, small, and round. Anisocytosis and anisokaryosis are mild, occasionally moderate.

2 What is your interpretation? What is the most likely origin of these cells? Cutaneous histiocytoma. This originates from Langerhans cells, which are epithelial dendritic cells with an antigen-presenting function.

3 What would be your therapeutic recommendation in the present case? Cutaneous histiocytoma is a common, benign, cutaneous tumor of the dog. Histiocytomas commonly occur as solitary lesions, which may undergo spontaneous regression within 2–3 months after onset. Monitoring is indicated and surgical excision with histopathologic examination is recommended, if regression does not occur. Recurrence is rare.

Editors' note: A common finding in aspirates from canine cutaneous histiocytoma is the presence of variable numbers of small lymphocytes (mostly cytotoxic T lymphocytes), which are a hallmark of ongoing tumor regression. These may become the predominant cell type and differentiation from a primary lymphoproliferative disease may be difficult. Cytochemical and inmunochemical techniques are available to confirm the origin of histiocytic cells, especially when cytology and/or histopathology alone are unable to provide a definitive diagnosis. Neoplastic cells in cutaneous histiocytoma are expected to be positive for E-cadherin, CD1a, CD11a/CD11c/CD18, CD44, CD45, and MHC class II. Tumor histiocytes variably express CD11b/CD18 and CD54.

Further reading
Moore PF (2014) A review of histiocytic diseases of dogs and cats. *Veterinary Pathology* **51**:167–184.

CASE 94

1 What cell(s) are increased in number in 94a? Plasma cells (1). These cells have moderate amounts of deeply basophilic cytoplasm and eccentric nuclei with a perinuclear clear area, which is the Golgi area, the site of immunoglobulin production. There also appears to be a mixed population of lymphoid cells with an increased percentage of large lymphoid cells (2).

2 What does this indicate? This indicates reactive lymphoid hyperplasia and particularly plasma cell hyperplasia.

3 What is the cell next to the arrowhead in 94b? A 'Mott cell'. This is a plasma cell containing Russell bodies, which are accumulations of immunoglobulins within vesicles.

4 Given the history and clinical signs, can you speculate on a possible cause for the generalized lymphadenopathy? Plasma cell hyperplasia is caused by chronic antigenic stimulation. In this case the cause was *Leishmania* infection. The organisms were identified in macrophages in a bone marrow aspirate.

Editors' note: Other cases in this book illustrate *Leishmania* organisms and lymphoid and plasma cell hyperplasia and Mott cells. This case is included to emphasize recognition of the basic processes and underlying mechanisms contributing to this cytologic appearance. Knowledge of the significance of the finding of hyperplasia, with the history of importation from Spain, indicated that additional investigation was required to identify the suspected organism. Other differential diagnoses for chronic immune stimulation that could result in this appearance cytologically include chronic parasitic, fungal, bacterial, or protozoal infections. Tick-borne diseases should be included in the differential in those countries or areas where tick exposure may be present. Sometimes, chronic, noninfectious disease processes, including neoplasia, systemic lupus erythematosus, or immune-mediated disease involving the skin and/or joints, could present with this appearance. Therefore, an extensive work up may be required in some cases in order to determine the most likely underlying cause. The cytologic evaluation is part of this work up.

CASE 95

1 Describe the cells identified. A cluster of cohesive nucleated cells is present. These cells show various degrees of anisokaryosis, a high N:C ratio, and prominent nucleoli. The chromatin pattern is particularly coarse. The round, pale staining area in the cytoplasm of the central cell is likely to reflect hydropic degeneration.

2 What is your provisional diagnosis? The adherent nature of the cells is consistent with epithelial origin and there are sufficient criteria to suggest malignancy. Given the body system affected and the cytologic features observed, transitional cell carcinoma is considered most likely.

3 What other tests may provide supportive evidence or definitive diagnosis? Double contrast radiographic studies or ultrasound examination may be useful, and in this case revealed a thickening of the dorsal bladder wall. The cytologic features are highly suggestive of neoplasia, but histologic examination of a biopsy may be required for a definitive diagnosis. In this case the histologic diagnosis confirmed a transitional cell carcinoma.

4 What prognosis is associated with this diagnosis? Transitional cell carcinoma has a guarded to poor prognosis. It may be multifocal, with some sites not apparent macroscopically. There is potential for metastasis, often to regional lymph nodes of the abdomen and pelvis, or to the long bones or pelvic bones.

Editors' note: A photomicrograph (95b; Papanicolaou, ×100 oil) from another dog with transitional cell carcinoma is included here for comparison. The smear contains small numbers of erythrocytes and many nucleated cells consistent with transitional epithelial origin, and showing marked cytologic features of atypia. These cells show moderate anisocytosis, with an increased N:C ratio. The nuclei are large and oval, with prominent chromatin clumping and some uneven thickening of nuclear membranes. One or more distinct nucleoli are often present. The cytoplasm varies from scant to moderately abundant and is granular to finely vacuolated. A few binucleated cells are seen. The nuclear details may be more easily evaluated with Hematoxylin staining (the nuclear stain used in the Papanicolaou stain) than with Romanowsky stains. The large cohesive group is the result of gentle traumatic exfoliation with a catheter in the area of a mass demonstrated radiographically. Individually exfoliated cells tend to 'round up' in the urine, while traumatically exfoliated groups more commonly appear as flat, cohesive groups of cells. This method of collection is beneficial in obtaining large numbers of cells for cytologic evaluation. The urine specimen was immediately fixed by the addition of two drops of 10% buffered formalin per ml of urine specimen. The fixation helps preserve cells during transport to the laboratory. Papanicolaou staining is not routinely available in commercial laboratories in North America, but is available at several laboratories in the UK and continental Europe. The use of various stains and fixatives varies, depending on pathologists' preference, experience, and training.

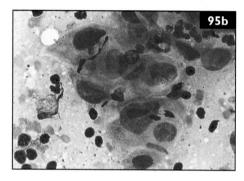

Answers

Further reading
Borjesson LL, Christopher MM, Ling GV (1999) Detection of canine transitional cell carcinoma using a bladder tumor antigen dipstick test. *Veterinary Clinical Pathology* **28**:33–38.
Roszel JF, Freeman KP (1988) Equine endometrial cytology. *Veterinary Clinics of North America (Equine)* **4(2)**, 247–262.

CASE 96

1 Describe the cells shown in the photomicrograph. The photomicrograph shows a mixed population of nucleated cells in a lightly basophilic background. There is a prevalence of neutrophils (frequently poorly preserved), with a lower percentage of lymphoid cells (orange arrow), mature plasma cells (green arrow), and a few macrophages (red arrow).

2 What are your differential diagnoses based on the history and these cytologic findings? These cytologic findings are consistent with a mixed, mostly neutrophilic lymphadenitis. Given the clinical history, juvenile cellulitis is considered likely.

'Puppy strangles', or juvenile cellulitis, is a nodular and pustular skin disorder that affects puppies. It usually occurs between the ages of 3 weeks and 4 months, and is rarely seen in adult dogs. Face, pinnae, and submandibular lymph nodes are the most common sites to be affected. The cause of this condition is unknown, but there are breeds that appear to be predisposed, including Golden Retrievers, Labrador Retrievers, and Dachshunds. The condition responds dramatically to corticosteroids, suggesting an immune dysfunction. Mixed lymphadenitis can also be observed in association with infectious diseases (e.g. fungi, *Mycobacterium*) and other less common conditions including vasculitis and hemosiderosis.

Further reading
White SD, Rosychuck RA, Stewart LK *et al.* (1989) Juvenile cellulitis in dogs: 15 cases. *Journal of the American Veterinary Medical Association* **195**:1609–1611.

CASE 97

1 Identify the cell population present in the smear, and describe the most relevant characteristics. On an abundant proteinaceous and eosinophilic background, there are large numbers of neutrophils exhibiting variable degenerative changes, including karyolysis (indicated by the arrows); in spite of these changes, no intracellular and/or extracellular bacteria are noted.

2 What is your final interpretation? Acute neutrophilic prostatitis – prostatic abscess. Acute prostatitis is usually suppurative and can arise at any age, but is more common in older dogs with prostatic hyperplasia and is uncommon in castrated dogs due to prostatic atrophy. Glandular changes associated with benign prostatic hyperplasia predispose to prostatic infection. Bacterial infection of the urinary tract in intact male dogs may spread to the prostate gland, usually as a result of ascension of normal aerobic urethral bacteria, or descend along the urethra from an infection in the urinary bladder. Septic prostatitis due to hematogenous dissemination of bacteria is also possible. *Escherichia coli* is the most commonly isolated organism in acute prostatitis, followed by *Staphylococcus aureus*, *Klebsiella* spp., *Proteus mirabilis*, *Mycoplasma canis*, *Pseudomonas aeruginosa*, and *Enterobacter* spp. Coalescing of focal areas of septic prostatitis may also result in prostatic abscesses and, in the absence of previous antibiotic therapy, intracellular and extracellular organisms may be seen.

An inflammatory leukogram characterized by peripheral neutrophilia, with or without a left-shift is a common finding, and frequent concurrent changes on blood chemistry panels (e.g. increase in acute phase proteins, hypoalbuminemia, hyperglobulinemia and hypoglycemia) may also be observed.

3 **What additional tests are recommended to confirm the hypothesis?** Microscopic examination and bacterial culture of the prostatic fluid. In this case, these tests confirmed the diagnosis of bacterial prostatitis.

CASE 98

1 **Describe the cytologic findings, and give your cytologic interpretation.** A population of round to spindle-shaped cells, either individual or forming small groups, is observed throughout the smear. These cells have a round to oval nucleus, granular chromatin, and prominent, round, single nucleoli. The cytoplasm is pale blue, variable in amount, and occasionally containing fine dusting black granules, consistent with melanin. These cells exhibit moderate anisocytosis and anisokaryosis and some binucleation. Rare small lymphocytes (indicated by the arrow) are also noted.

The presence of a population of atypical nucleated cells, occasionally containing melanin, in a lymph node aspirate is consistent with metastatic melanoma.

Preoperative cytologic evaluation of FNAs of regional lymph nodes, regardless of their size, is useful for clinical staging and it is always strongly encouraged. A previous study on the association between lymph node size and metastasis in dogs with oral malignant melanoma showed that of all dogs with cytologic or histologic evidence of mandibular lymph node metastasis, up to one-third had mandibular lymph nodes of normal size.

Further reading
Herring ES, Smith MM, Robertson JL (2002) Lymph node staging of oral and maxillofacial neoplasms in 31 dogs and cats. *Journal of Veterinary Dentistry* **19**:122–126.

Answers

Kerr ME, Burgess HJ (2013) What is your diagnosis? Gingival mass in a dog. *Veterinary Clinical Pathology* **42**:116–117.

Williams LE, Packer RA (2003) Association between lymph node size and metastasis in dogs with oral malignant melanoma: 100 cases (1987–2001). *Journal of the American Veterinary Medical Association* **222**:1234–1236.

CASE 99

1 Examine the nuclei – are there any criteria of malignancy? The nuclei are quite large with stippled chromatin and many have prominent nucleoli. Some cells have a single, large, fairly central nucleolus. Others have two or multiple nucleoli (1). The N:C ratio is increased.

2 Examine the cytoplasm – are there granules present? A few cells have dark green/black intracytoplasmic granules – these are melanin granules (2).

3 What is your interpretation? Melanocytic tumor. Given the anatomic location, paucity of melanin granules, and the nuclear features of atypia, the tumor is likely malignant (melanoma). These tumors often metastasize to local and distant sites, so the prognosis is guarded.

4 What would you do next? Tumor staging is required before treatment. Local lymph nodes should be palpated and aspirated, regardless of size. A previous study showed that over 30% of dogs with proven cytologic or histologic evidence of lymph node metastases of melanoma had lymph nodes of normal size. Chest radiographs should also be taken to rule out pulmonary metastasis.

Further reading
Williams LE, Packer RA (2003) Association between lymph node size and metastasis in dogs with oral malignant melanoma: 100 cases (1987–2001). *Journal of the American Veterinary Medical Association* **222**(9):1234–1236.

CASE 100

1 Describe the background of the smear. There is a large amount of golden-brown granular material present. This is bile pigment, which may be intracellular or extracellular. It can vary in color from golden-brown to blue–green or purple–gray.

2 Identify the cells present. There is a mixed population of macrophages and degenerate neutrophils. However, in this case a delay in preparation of smears of the fluid may have contributed to the loss of neutrophil nuclear integrity.

3 What is your provisional diagnosis, and what other tests may be used to confirm this diagnosis? The gross appearance of the fluid and the cytologic features are typical of a biliary peritonitis. The cellular response in such cases is very variable, but the presence of bile usually results in an inflammatory response. Comparison of the bilirubin concentration in the serum and fluid may aid in the diagnosis. The fluid may be sterile or septic. No bacteria were isolated in this case and the trauma to the common bile duct was repaired surgically. The patient made an uneventful recovery.

Editors' note: Bile pigment may range from golden-brown to yellow or blue–green or purple–gray in Wright–Giemsa and Papanicolaou-stained smears of bilious effusions. In some smears it may have a granular purple appearance and it may be difficult to distinguish unless there is some green to golden-brown material that suggests bile pigment. It may vary in amount, depending on the degree of damage, amount of bile leakage, and duration of the condition. Because it is noncellular, bile pigment may be easily overlooked if not present in large amounts, or confused with other sources of pigment or precipitate, such as hemorrhage. Correct identification and recognition of its significance provide valuable information that can initiate additional confirmatory testing and thus provide a timely assessment before attempts to repair the underlying damage to the biliary system.

CASE 101

1 **Identify the cell population present in the smear and describe the most relevant characteristics.** The samples are hypercellular and contain a population of pleomorphic large round cells. The cytoplasm is moderate, slightly basophilic, and granular. Nuclei are round to cerebroid, central to eccentric, with fine reticular chromatin and prominent round nucleoli. Cellular atypia is moderate, and frequent mitotic figures are seen.

2 **What differential diagnoses would you consider?** These cytologic findings are supportive of a malignant 'round cell' tumor. Differential diagnoses include a neoplasia of either histiocytic or lymphoid origin. Based on the location, a poorly differentiated amelanotic melanoma also should be included in the differential list.

3 **What additional tests might be recommended?** Since a definitive cytologic diagnosis could not be reached on the basis of routine cytologic examination alone, histology and immunohistochemistry would be advisable to further investigate the origin of these neoplastic cells. Immunohistiochemistry was performed for the following markers: CD3 (pan T-cell marker), CD20/CD79a (B-cell markers), MUM1 (plasma cell marker), CD18 (histiocytic and lymphoid marker), and Melan A (melanocyte marker). Melan A was positive and a final diagnosis of poorly pigmented malignant melanoma was made. Metastasis to the submandibular lymph node was identified on regional lymph node aspirates.

Further reading
Przeździecki R, Czopowicz M, Sapierzyński R (2015) Accuracy of routine cytology and immunocytochemistry in preoperative diagnosis of oral amelanotic melanomas in dogs. *Veterinary Clinical Pathology* **44**:597–604.

CASE 102

1 What is the cytologic interpretation of this CSF? There is a markedly increased number of inflammatory cells (pleocytosis). These cells predominantly consist of small lymphocytes (>60%) and large mononuclear cells, likely macrophages. No bacterial or other infectious agents can be seen.

2 What are the possible differential diagnoses? Mononuclear pleocytosis can be associated with viral (e.g. distemper, rabies), protozoal (e.g. *Toxoplasma, Neospora*) or fungal infections, meningitis of unknown origin (MEUO), or neoplasia (e.g. lymphoma), as well as less common causes such as uremia, vaccine reaction, or diskospondylitis. Given the clinical history and signalment and absence of findings suggestive of infection, a diagnosis of MEUO is most likely, although serology and/or PCR testing are recommended to rule out *Toxoplasma* or *Neospora* infection. Canine distemper virus or rabies are both unlikely given that the dog was vaccinated.

CASE 103

1 What are the structures indicated by the arrows? There is a clump of filamentous gram-negative rods.

2 List two organisms that have this kind of morphology. *Actinomyces* species and *Nocardia* species are bacterial genera that have similar morphology. Of the two, *Actinomyces* is most likely in cases of pyothorax in the cat.

3 How can you differentiate between the two before culture results can be received? An acid-fast stain (either Ziehl–Neelsen or Kinyoun's Cold Acid-Fast) would differentiate the two species; *Nocardia* species are variably positive for acid-fast stain, while *Actinomyces* are acid-fast negative.

CASE 104

1 What is the most likely diagnosis? The signalment, history, palpation, imaging, and cytologic observations are most compatible with transitional cell carcinoma, the most common bladder neoplasm in the dog. Cytologic key features include: cells that are found singly or in aggregates, marked anisocytosis and anisokaryosis, presence of cytoplasmic vacuoles in some cells, variable cytoplasmic basophilia and N:C ratios, and pink globular intracytoplasmic inclusions (not seen in the picture).

Editors' note: Transitional cell carcinoma may be a difficult diagnosis in cases with extensive hemorrhage and/or inflammation and atypical cells associated with irritation and whose features may mimic malignancy. Degeneration of cells may further complicate evaluation for features of malignancy. The most useful cytologic specimens usually are obtained by ultrasound-guided aspiration or gentle washing and gentle catheter trauma in the area of the mass.

Collection of specimens other than the first urine in the morning may be of benefit in obtaining cells with less degeneration. Gentle catheter trauma in the area of a mass that has been demonstrated by radiography and/or ultrasound may be helpful in obtaining large numbers of cells. Fixation immediately in an approximately equal volume of cold 40–50% ethanol or addition of two drops of 10% buffered formalin per ml of specimen, followed by refrigeration prior to submission to the laboratory, is helpful in preserving cellular morphology when Papanicolaou staining is available. If Papanicolaou staining is not available and Romanowsky staining is, preparation of an air-dried smear from sediment from a freshly collected specimen is recommended. Refrigeration of the urine specimen is of benefit in preserving cellular morphology if the specimen cannot be processed immediately.

CASE 105

1 What are the structures seen in the smear, and what are they called? The aspirate is characterized by numerous anucleated squamous epithelial cells ('ghost cells', because of their characteristic appearance with a central, small and round empty zone). Keratinized anucleated squamous epithelial cells without the characteristic central clear area are simply known as 'squames.'

2 What are your main differential diagnoses? These cytologic findings indicate aspiration from a keratinized lesion. Moreover, the presence of numerous ghost cells is consistent with pilomatricoma. Pilomatricoma is an uncommon benign tumor that arises from the germinative cells of the hair bulb. Ghost cells indicate a hair follicle origin, and form during the process of matrical keratinization of the neoplastic population. During this process, the accumulation of a large amount of keratin in cytoplasm causes the degeneration of the nucleus, leading to the formation of the typical empty zone. Although ghost cells are most frequently seen in pilomatricomas, their presence is not pathognomonic, as they can be found in other cutaneous tumors such as trichoepitheliomas and follicular cysts. Malignant pilomatricomas have only rarely been reported in dogs.

Further reading
Jackson K, Boger L, Goldschmidt M *et al.* (2010) Malignant pilomatricoma in a soft-coated Wheaten Terrier. *Veterinary Clinical Pathology* **39**:236–240.
Masserdotti C, Ubbiali FM (2002) Fine needle aspiration cytology of pilomatricoma in three dogs. *Veterinary Clinical Pathology* **31**:22–25.

Answers

CASE 106

1 Describe the cells seen in the photomicrograph. The smear is highly cellular and is characterized by a cluster of well-differentiated hepatocytes (in the center of the photomicrograph), with biliary casts (extra hepatic cholestasis). Around this, there is a population of discrete round cells, likely lymphoid in origin, with moderate amounts of lightly basophilic cytoplasm and round, frequently indented and lobulated nuclei, with irregularly clumped chromatin and small round nucleoli.

2 What is your interpretation? Round cell neoplasia, suggestive of hepatic lymphoma. A round cell tumor of other origin (e.g. histiocytic) is considered a less likely differential. The presence of marked hyperbilirubinemia in the peripheral blood and biliary casts on liver cytology suggest obstruction of biliary outflow.

3 What additional tests might be useful in order to stage the disease? As part of the clinical staging, a complete evaluation of peripheral and visceral lymph nodes and spleen are recommended. Bone marrow examination should also be considered, especially in the presence of peripheral cytopenias and/or atypical circulating cells; this will help to rule out a possible leukemic phase. Hepatic lymphoma may occur as a primary lesion or be part of a systemic process (multicentric lymphoma). A complete clinical staging and immunophenotype analysis are both important steps in the therapeutic and prognostic management.

CASE 107

Identify the exogenous and possible foreign body material in the photomicrograph (107; Wright Giemsa, ×100 oil). The photomicrograph shows granular stain precipitate that forms as the dye oxidizes and crystallizes, potentially mimicking bacterial cocci or *Mycoplasma* but more irregular, nondividing, and more refractile. This underlines the importance of changing stains frequently in order to avoid formation of precipitate products and bacterial contamination, which may hamper a correct interpretation of the sample.

CASE 108

1 What is the organism shown? *Demodex canis*, the causative agent of so-called 'red mange' (demodicosis).

2 Why is it important to see multiple life stages? It is important to see multiple life stages to confirm active proliferation consistent with infection. This follicular mite can also sometimes be found in skin scrapings of asymptomatic dogs. Multiple life stages as seen here indicate active proliferation. The adults have eight legs, the nymphs have six legs, and the bodies are elongate.

CASE 109

1 What cells are present? The smears are filled with reactive macrophages and lymphocytes, together with occasional neutrophils and disrupted cells. The outline of nonstaining or lightly staining rod-shaped organisms can be seen in a macrophage in **109c**. A few extracellular organisms are present.

2 What is your interpretation? Granulomatous inflammation. Subsequently, tissue from a surgical biopsy stained positively for mycobacterial organisms with Ziehl–Neelsen (acid-fast) stain, and a diagnosis of feline mycobacteriosis was made.

Editors' note: If granulomatous inflammation is identified in a cat, mycobacterial infection should be part of the differential diagnosis. Careful scrutiny of smears and tissue sections may be needed to detect intracytoplasmic organisms, and additional investigation by Ziehl–Neelsen staining of aspirates and tissue sections should be pursued. Additional tests, such as PCR, may be needed to demonstrate infection when organisms are few.

CASE 110

1 What are the structures seen on the photomicrograph? The structures are consistent with hyaline casts.

2 How can their visibility be improved? Hyaline casts are highly translucent and nonrefractory casts. They are easier to identify in a fresh urine sample, instead of stored samples. To improve their visibility, it is recommended to lower the condenser, dim the light, and screen the sediment at low magnification (×10 or ×20). Casts can also be stained by mixing a drop of sediment with a drop of 0.5% New Methylene Blue in saline.

3 Explain how those structures likely formed in this case. Casts consist of gelatinous Tamm–Horsfall mucoprotein. They are unstable and deteriorate in dilute urine and/or alkaline pH. Casts are always renal in origin. Cast formation usually takes place in the distal and collecting tubules. In this patient the poor renal perfusion caused by dehydration, with subsequent diuresis, most likely caused the cylindruria.

Editors' note: Hyaline casts are often associated with the presence of proteinuria. In such cases, it has been proposed that the presence of excessive serum protein in the tubular lumen may promote the precipitation of the Tamm–Horsfall mucoprotein.

Further reading
Mundt LA, Shanahan K (2010) *Graff's Textbook of Urinalysis and Body Fluids*. Lippincott Williams & Wilkins, Philadelphia.

Answers

CASE 111

1 Identify the cell populations present, and describe the other features in this field.
Highly vacuolated macrophages and neutrophils are present. The latter are seen more readily at the higher magnification. Note the round to oval structures with blue/purple central region, a clear thick halo, and very variable size.

2 Classify the inflammatory response present. Does this provide any help with regard to the origin of the structures present in this field? There is evidence of a mixed (macrophagic and neutrophilic) inflammatory response, which may be associated with fungal infection, mycobacterial infection, foreign body, panniculitis, or protozoal infection. Sometimes pyogranulomatous inflammation is also seen with reactions to foreign bodies or penetrating wounds or reactions to tick, insect, or spider bites. The structures present are consistent with fungal infection due to *Cryptococcus* species. Differentiation of several species of *Cryptococcus* may require additional testing.

3 What is your provisional diagnosis, and how might this be confirmed? The presence of a mixed inflammatory response with variably sized organisms with a clear halo is consistent with a fungal infection. Culture of material from the lesion produced a profuse growth of *C. neoformans*. Cryptococcosis can produce subcutaneous swellings, although it is more commonly associated with respiratory tract or neurologic disease. The cellular response associated with infection is variable and, as in this case, the number of organisms may appear greater than the number of inflammatory cells. Cryptococcosis more commonly affects cats than dogs. The prognosis for feline cryptococcosis appears to have been improved by the use of fluconazole, but the owner of this cat requested euthanasia.

CASE 112

1 What cells and structures can you identify in the photomicrograph? There are scattered neutrophils, some of which are outside the plane of focus. There are two large, orange–pink cells with central, small, oval nuclei that are squamous epithelial cells and consistent with oropharyngeal origin. The orange–pink staining of squamous epithelium with the Papanicolaou stain is indicative of the presence of keratohyalin and its precursors. Some small bacterial rods are present in clumps in the center and upper left.

2 Other fields in the cytologic preparation failed to demonstrate any macrophages or columnar or cuboidal epithelial cells. The features in the photomicrograph are representative of the entire smear. What is your conclusion? In the absence of cells representative of the pulmonary tree (macrophages and columnar or cuboidal epithelial cells), the specimen likely reflects oropharyngeal contamination. The neutrophils may reflect oropharyngeal inflammation. Therefore, the cytologic specimen is considered unsatisfactory for evaluation since it lacks cells representative of the lung. Some macrophages and epithelial cells from large (columnar) and/or small airways (cuboidal epithelium and/or macrophages) should be present for tracheal washing to be considered satisfactory for evaluation and likely to be representative of the lung.

Oropharyngeal contamination is more likely to occur if the horse is fractious, if the mouth is not washed out prior to collection, or if the passage of the endoscope into the trachea is difficult or prolonged. A note to the cytologist indicating whether any of these events has occurred is often helpful in determining if such cells are likely to be due to contamination. If cells representative of the lung are present and oropharyngeal material is also seen, the possibility of oropharyngeal contamination or of abnormal drainage of oropharyngeal material into the trachea in association with a laryngeal or pharyngeal abnormality should be considered. A small amount of oropharyngeal material may be considered to be within expected limits for background contamination. There are skilled collectors who seldom submit endoscopic washings with evidence of oropharyngeal contamination. When oropharyngeal material is present in their specimens, the author always cautions them to consider possible laryngeal or pharyngeal dysfunction in their differential diagnoses. Dynamic evaluation of oropharyngeal and laryngeal function with exercise on the treadmill may be needed in order to diagnosis pharyngeal or laryngeal dysfunction that may contribute to oropharyngeal material draining into the trachea and/or bronchi in some cases.

CASE 113

1 Identify the cell population present in the smears, and describe the most relevant characteristics. Samples are hypercellular, containing epithelial cells arranged in variably sized sheets and clusters with a characteristic honeycomb pattern on a hemorrhagic background. Occasionally, acinar-like arrangement is noted and cytoplasmic borders appear indistinct. The cells are relatively uniform in appearance, with a low to moderate N:C ratio and a moderately basophilic cytoplasm. The cytoplasm is slightly granular in appearance, and sometimes vacuolated. Nuclei are round to oval, variably central to eccentrically located, displaying mild anisokaryosis, with fine chromatin pattern and inconspicuous nucleoli. Occasionally, clusters of cuboidal cells with an increased N:C ratio are seen. The columnar nature of the cells is most easily appreciated at the edges of the groups, where basal nuclear position is seen and the cytoplasm can be identified in profile, while the honeycomb or mosaic appearance of the epithelium is most easily appreciated in the central areas of the groups where cells are seen on end. These findings help differentiate simple columnar to cuboidal epithelium of prostatic gland origin from the multilayered epithelium more typical of transitional epithelium, which frequently has more central nuclei and more varied cytoplasmic shape.

2 What is your final interpretation? Benign prostatic hyperplasia (BPH). BPH is the most common prostatic disorder in the dog and is mainly observed in intact adult male dogs as a result of androgenic stimulation. Clinical signs may be absent, although tenesmus, persistent or intermittent hematuria, and dysuria may be observed.

3 What are the different methods for collecting cytologic samples from the prostate gland? Material from prostatic gland can be obtained most reliably from ultrasound-guided aspirates from the gland. Sometimes, material representative of the prostate can be obtained directly through the urethra with or without prostatic massage, although most often the material retrieved reflects urinary tract and transitional epithelial origin. Washing the part of the urethra near the prostate with a few milliliters of saline, through delicate injection and aspiration, and gently massaging the prostate may help to obtain more cellular and representative samples when a urinary catheter is used.

CASE 114

1 Describe the cells shown in the photomicrograph. The background is clear with small numbers of RBCs and cellular debris. There is a main population of small lymphoid cells; these often appear elongated with small amounts of pale blue, basophilic cytoplasm that is often elongated at one pole of the nucleus. Some have a distinctive linear elongation resembling a handle (hand-mirror cells). Nuclei are round, slightly angular or elongated, small, and eccentrically located, with condensed chromatin and indistinct nucleoli.

2 What is your interpretation? The presence of a monomorphic population of small lymphoid cells in a sample from an enlarged lymph node is primarily supportive of small cell lymphoma. Moreover, some of cytologic features (e.g. hand-mirror cells) are suggestive of a low-grade T-cell form (small clear cell/T-zone lymphoma). The presence of lymphoma is further supported by the peripheral lymphocytosis, which is often observed in cases of small clear cell/T-zone lymphoma and indicates spread of the neoplastic process to the peripheral blood and likely bone marrow (stage V lymphoma). Paracortical hyperplasia is another possible differential diagnosis. When small cell lymphoma is suspected, further investigations are needed for a definitive diagnosis and prior to treatment.

3 What further tests would you recommend to reach a definitive diagnosis? Flow cytometric immunophenotyping is strongly recommended in these cases and will help to confirm and further characterize the process. In small clear cell/T-zone lymphoma, neoplastic cells commonly exhibit a characteristic aberrant immunophenotype with lack of CD45 (panleukocytic marker) and frequently an aberrant expression of CD21 (B-lymphoid marker), together with a classical positivity to T-cell markers (CD5, CD3, frequently CD4+ and/or CD8+). PARR on the prestained smears also may be useful in confirming the monoclonal proliferation supportive of lymphoid neoplasia and demonstrating the T-cell origin of these cells. Histopathology may also help solve differentials. In this case it showed marked expansion of the paracortical area and effacement of the normal lymph node architecture. This type of lymphoma typically exhibits slowly progressive indolent biological behavior. The median survival time varies among studies, but is generally reported as months to years.

Further reading
Martini V, Marconato L, Poggi A *et al.* (2015) Canine small clear cell/T-zone lymphoma: clinical presentation and outcome in a retrospective case series. *Veterinary Comparative Oncology* **14(Suppl 1)**:117–126.
Martini V, Poggi A, Riondato F *et al.* (2015) Flow-cytometric detection of phenotypic aberrancies in canine small clear cell lymphoma. *Veterinary Comparative Oncology* **13**:281–287.
Seelig DM, Avery P, Webb T *et al.* (2014) Canine T-zone lymphoma: unique immunophenotypic features, outcome, and population characteristics. *Journal of Internal Medicine* **28**:878–888.

CASE 115

1 How would you describe the wash, and what are the coiled structures in 115a? Mixed inflammation (pneumonia) with evidence of chronic (resolving) active hemorrhage. The kinetics of the hemorrhage can be determined due to the presence of platelets (active) and hemosiderin (chronic) (seen in other fields of view). The coiled structures are first-stage parasitic larvae <200 microns in length.
2 At higher magnification these larvae demonstrate kinked tails (115b). What are the most likely differentials in dogs? If similar larvae were identified in cats, what is the most likely differential? *Filaroides* species (*Oslerus osleri* and *Filaroides hirthi*), *Angiostrongylus vasorum* or *Crenosoma vulpis* in a dog; *Aleurostrongylus abstrusus* in a cat.
3 Is an intermediate host required in the life cycle of *Filaroides* species? If so, name the species, and if not, comment why. No intermediate host is required, since *Filaroides* species are directly infective as first-stage larvae, and development through all five stages is completed in the lung tissue of the dog. Infection is acquired through the ingestion of regurgitated stomach contents, lung tissue, or feces of infected dogs. Autoinfection can thus worsen the worm burden within an animal.

4 How would you confirm the diagnosis? Fecal specimens, using zinc sulfate flotation or Baermann technique to identify the larvae. An ELISA antigen test for *Angiostrongylus vasorum* is also available.

Editors' note: Filaroid worms in dogs have been reported in many countries, including the USA, UK, South Africa, New Zealand, France, and Australia. They vary in length from 5 mm to 15 mm. If endoscopy is used for collection of a respiratory cytology specimen and evaluation of the respiratory tract, nodules in the area of the distal trachea or area of bifurcation of the major bronchi are classically associated with *O. osleri*. *F. hirthi* occurs in the lung parenchyma. The bitch may transfer larvae in its saliva to puppies. Following ingestion, larvae are carried by blood to the lungs.

    A. vasorum is a relatively common lungworm in the UK. It has a snail intermediate host and may present with coagulopathy, particularly bleeding into the lung. It is reported to be common in racing Greyhounds, but may be seen in a variety of working and pet dogs.

    Cytology is best for diagnosis of *F. hirthi*, but low-grade infections may not produce sufficient larvae to be detected. Either zinc sulfate flotation or a Baermann technique may be useful in demonstrating larvae.

Further reading
Ettinger SJ, Feldman EC (2010) *Textbook of Veterinary Internal Medicine*, 7th edn. WB Saunders, Philadelphia.
Fisher M (2001) Endoparasites in the dog and cat. *In Practice* **23**(8):462–471.
Wright D, Bauman D (1999) *Georgis' Parasitology for Veterinarians*, 7th edn. WB Saunders, Philadelphia, pp. 187–191.

CASE 116

1 What is the structure in the central right portion of the photomicrograph? A corpus amylacea. This is an acellular structure that could be confused with a cell since it has a densely staining center that can be mistaken for a nucleus. The peripheral, concentric layers are less dense and should not be confused with cytoplasm. These bodies are thought to be composed of glycoproteins and they do not calcify. They are found in respiratory cytology specimens in humans with chronic alveolar edema and/or obstruction due to cardiac insufficiency, pulmonary infarction, and chronic bronchitis. They may be seen in low numbers in respiratory specimens from horses, dogs, and cats with similar conditions.

2 What is its significance in a respiratory cytology specimen? The corpus amylacea is significant since it supports the history of chronic obstruction. Casts of inspissated mucus with many embedded neutrophils were seen in other fields of this tracheal washing smear and provided additional cytologic support for mechanical obstruction of airways.

CASE 117

1 Describe the cells shown in the three photomicrographs. There are high numbers of erythrocytes and neutrophils, and nucleated cells with features of malignancy. The latter occur singly and in cohesive groups, some with papillary configuration. These cells have oval, paracentral nuclei with coarse granular chromatin and prominent round nucleoli. The cytoplasm is moderate, basophilic, and varies from homogeneous to finely vacuolated.

2 What is your interpretation of these findings? The cytologic features are consistent with an epithelial neoplasm, likely pulmonary adenocarcinoma. The possibility of a metastatic tumor that has broken through from the interstitium into the airway lumen cannot be completely ruled out, but the degree of cellularity is high and a primary pulmonary malignancy is most likely.

3 What comment would you make about this condition? Pulmonary adenocarcinoma often has metastases to other areas of the lung through blood vessels, lymphatics, or airways. Bronchial lymph nodes are also often involved.

CASE 118

Identify the exogenous and possible foreign body material in this photomicrograph (118; Wright–Giemsa, ×20). The photomicrograph shows granular magenta gel precipitate, likely ultrasound gel, which may completely obscure any cellular harvest. Ultrasound-guided sampling should occur after removal of the gel from the skin, using an alcohol-based liquid instead as the sonographic medium for contact.

CASE 119

1 Describe the cytologic findings in photomicrograph 119a. The sample is highly cellular with adequate preservation. The background is clear with frequent lymphoglandular bodies and a few bare nuclei. There is a main population of pleomorphic, medium, and large lymphoid cells. These have scarce, deeply blue cytoplasm and a clear perinuclear halo is frequently seen. Nuclei are large in size (diameter >2 RBCs), round, with poorly condensed chromatin. One to multiple, prominent, round nucleoli are frequently seen. Three mitotic figures are identifiable in the center of the image, together with several disrupted cells probably of the same origin of the blast cells described above.

2 What is your interpretation? High-grade lymphoma.

3 What cells are shown in photomicrograph 119b, and what is the likely immunophenotype? Large lymphoid cells with prominent nucleoli, likely neoplastic centroblasts and immunoblasts (1). Intermediate sized lymphoid cells with a single, central, prominent nucleoli, likely medium-sized macronucleolated cells from the marginal zone (2). An admixed population of neoplastic centroblasts and medium sized macronucleolated cells, together with high mitotic activity, are all characteristic of high-grade B-cell lymphoma (centroblastic pleomorphic type). From a histologic point this corresponds to a diffuse large B-cell lymphoma subtype, the most common canine lymphoma subtype. Immunophenotyping via flow cytometry, immunocytochemistry, or immunohistochemistry showed positivity to B-cell markers (CD21, CD79a, CD20, surface immunoglobulins).

Further reading
Fournel-Fleury C, Magnol JP, Bricaire P et al. (1997) Cytohistological and immunological classification of canine malignant lymphomas: comparison with human non-Hodgkin's lymphomas. *Journal of Comparative Pathology* **117**:35–59.
Ponce F, Marchal T, Magnol JP et al. (2010) A morphological study of 608 cases of canine malignant lymphoma in France with a focus on comparative similarities between canine and human lymphoma morphology. *Veterinary Pathology* **47**:414–433.

CASE 120
1 The cells in the photomicrograph are most consistent with what general cell lineage? The formation of loose to densely disorganized groups and the spindloid shape of the cells characterized by indistinct cell margins are most consistent with a lesion of mesenchymal origin.

2 Do these cells exhibit cytologic criteria of malignancy? What is your cytologic interpretation? These cells exhibit moderate criteria of malignancy, including moderate anisocytosis and anisokaryosis, nuclear pleomorphism, and multiple nucleoli. The cytologic diagnosis is soft tissue sarcoma. Based on the location and cytologic appearance, peripheral nerve sheath tumor is a likely differential diagnosis; however, cytology cannot reliably subclassify different types of soft tissue sarcoma. Histopathology confirmed the diagnosis of a grade 1 peripheral nerve sheath tumor.

3 What is the most likely biological behavior of this type of lesion? These types of lesions tend to be locally aggressive but metastasis is uncommon. Unfortunately, in this case the lesion did extend to the surgical margins, increasing the chances of local recurrence. The tumor did eventually recur and required a second wider excision.

CASE 121
1 Identify the cells labeled 1, 2, and 3 in 121a. Provide an overall interpretation, and explain the significance of these cells within your interpretation. Mast cell tumor (MCT) with secondary eosinophils and fibrocyte proliferation. The significance

of the individual cells is as follows: 1 = eosinophils: mast cells release eosinophil chemotactic factor, IL3, IL5, and GM-CSF, which attract eosinophils. The precise role of eosinophils in MCTs is as yet undetermined. 2 = fibrocytes/fibroblasts: these are often seen in MCTs, since mast cells release chemokines that attract fibrocytes to the tumor location. In a histology section the presence of a fibrocyte component is seen as varying amounts of fibrous connective tissue around the neoplastic mast cells. 3 = mast cells.

Mast cell granules contain an impressive array of physiologically active chemical mediators, the two most important being histamine and heparin, the latter imparting the purple–red (metachromatic) color to the granules. Histamine and heparin pose risks in that histamine can result in severe intraoperative hypertension and heparin in some MCTs can be associated with coagulopathy/hemorrhage.

2 What is the prognosis for the tumor represented in 121a compared with 121b?
MCTs vary in biological activity but all tumors should be considered to be at least potentially malignant. They can be histologically graded using a system developed by Patnaik (in 1984), based primarily on nuclear morphology and localization within epidermal/dermal and subcutaneous tissue. This system appears to correlate with the clinical outcome, with grade I tumors usually carrying a favorable prognosis and grade III tumors typically associated with a guarded prognosis. The biological behavior of grade II tumors remains difficult to predict with this system. **121a** was histologically confirmed as a grade I tumor and **121b** was a grade III tumor. Note how rare the mast cell granules are and the bizarre neoplastic cytologic features in the grade III tumor. A 2-tier histologic grading system has been recently published by Kiupel in order to improve concordance among pathologists and to provide more accurate prognostication. According to this novel grading system, high-grade MCTs were significantly associated with shorter time to metastasis or new tumor development, and with shorter survival time. The median survival time was <4 months for high-grade MCTs but >2 years for low-grade MCTs.

3 Why is it important to aspirate/biopsy the local lymph node in a confirmed mast cell tumor? Regional lymph nodes are the site of highest frequency of metastasis.

Editors' note: 121b illustrates well a feature that may be useful in increasing the index of suspicion for MCT in cases with poor differentiation and few granules. Note the multiple small cytoplasmic vacuoles and the fact that some of these appear to extend across the nucleus. These are hypothesized to represent spaces where granules may have been previously. They differ from vacuoles seen with secretion and adenocarcinoma based on their small size and apparent extension across the nucleus. They do not stain positively for mucus with Mucicarmine or PAS stains.

Answers

Further reading
Gross TL, Ihrke PJ, Walder J (1992) (eds) *Veterinary Dermatohistopathology: A Macroscopic and Microscopic Evaluation of Canine and Feline Skin Disease*. Mosby, St. Louis, pp. 470–473.
Kiupel M, Webster JD, Bailey KL *et al.* (2011) Proposal of a 2-tier histologic grading system for canine cutaneous mast cell tumors to more accurately predict biological behavior. *Veterinary Pathology* **48**(1):147–155.
Yager JA, Wilcock JP (1994) Tumors of the skin and associated tissues. In: *Color Atlas and Text of Surgical Pathology of the Dog and Cat: Dermatopathology and Skin Tumors.* (eds. JA Yager, JP Wilcock). Mosby, London, pp. 278–279.

CASE 122

1 What are the cells seen in this photomicrograph, and what is the overall interpretation of this sample? Surface epithelial cells. This general term is used to describe cells, including meningeal, choroid plexus, ependymal, and endothelial cells, that may be found in CSF samples and are difficult to distinguish cytologically. These cells frequently form small clusters. Their morphology may vary from cuboidal to columnar or ovoid; basophilic faintly granular cytoplasm is common. The CSF characteristics in this case are unremarkable, with no evidence of pleocytosis and no increase in protein.

2 What is their significance in a CSF specimen? The presence of surface epithelial cells is an incidental finding in CSF and without clinical significance. Previous studies have not identified any association with age, disease type, nucleated cell count, or protein concentration. All diagnostic investigations performed (including neurologic imaging) were unremarkable, and idiopathic epilepsy was suspected.

Further reading
Wessmann A, Volk HA, Chandler K *et al.* (2010) Significance of surface epithelial cells in canine cerebrospinal fluid and relationship to central nervous system disease. *Veterinary Clinical Pathology* **39**:358–364.

CASE 123

1 What is your interpretation? The location of the lesion, the concurrent presence of a similar lesion on the tongue, and the cytologic observations are compatible with an indolent ulcer. This lesion forms part of the eosinophilic granuloma complex (EGC). Other lesions in this complex include the eosinophilic granuloma or linear granuloma and eosinophilic plaque, all cutaneous or mucocutaneous lesions found in cats. There is a possible link to allergens with these lesions, and for this reason the environment should be checked for possible allergens (e.g. flea bite sensitivity, food allergy, and/or atopy).

Editors' note: The cytologic finding of mixed inflammation, including eosinophils, is not specific for eosinophilic plaque/granuloma complex but, in conjunction with the clinical appearance of the lesion, supports this diagnosis. Differential diagnoses for this type of inflammation include reactions to foreign bodies and insect or spider bites or other types of bite wounds, fungal infections, or fly irritation. Aspirates are recommended rather than impression smears from the surface of lesions since this type of inflammation may be seen with ulcerated skin and/or mucocutaneous tumors, and impression smears may not provide the variety of cells that occur deeper in the tissue.

CASE 124

1 **Describe the cells shown in the photomicrograph.** There is a main population of highly pleomorphic large round cells, often bi- or multinucleated, with abundant, basophilic, often microvacuolated cytoplasm, sometimes showing characteristic cytoplasmic blebs (1). Nuclei are single or multiple, round, centrally to paracentrally located, with poorly condensed chromatin and occasional visible round nucleoli. Several criteria of malignancy are noted, including moderate anisocytosis, anisokaryosis, and multinucleation. A few residual small lymphocytes are also seen (2).

2 **What is your interpretation?** Metastatic 'round cell' tumor. Lymphoid tissue is almost completely effaced by the neoplastic population and only occasional residual small lymphocytes are seen. Differential diagnoses include acute myeloid leukemia (likely megakaryoblastic type, AML-M7), disseminated histiocytic sarcoma, and anaplastic lymphoma. The concurrent presence of some typical cytologic features, including round nuclei, cytoplasmic blebs, and vacuolization, is supportive of an acute megakaryoblastic leukemia.

Immunocytochemistry was performed and the cells were positive to platelet antigen Factor VIII, CD41, and CD61, confirming a megakaryocytic origin. Similar neoplastic cells were also identified in the peripheral blood, together with several large cytoplasmic fragments, resembling giant platelets, and in the bone marrow. Anemia and thrombocytopenia were also present. Similar to all the other acute myeloid leukemia subtypes, the prognosis is very poor. The response to chemotherapy is also consistently poor.

Further reading
Comazzi S, Gelain ME, Bonfanti U et al. (2010) Acute megakaryoblastic leukemia in dogs: a report of three cases and review of the literature. *Journal of the American Animal Hospital Association* 46:327–335.

CASE 125

1 Describe the cells shown in the photomicrograph. What is the likely tissue origin of these cells? There are frequent round cells with uniform round nuclei, abundant pink–purple cytoplasm, and variably sized, discrete, clear vacuoles. These cells are characteristic of brown fat and are often mistaken for epithelioid macrophages or glandular epithelium on cytology.

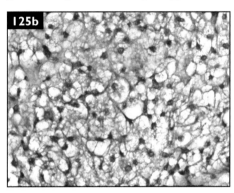

2 Is the lesion inflammatory or neoplastic? Neoplastic. Histology was performed and showed variably vacuolated round to polygonal cells, forming small packets supported by vascular fibrous connective tissue and confirming a diagnosis of hibernoma (125b; H&E, ×60). Confirmation of brown fat origin requires immunohistochemical staining with UPC 1 (uncoupling protein 1), Myogenin, Myo D, and Myf5.

Further reading
Ravi M, Schobert CS, Kiupel M et al. (2014) Clinical, morphologic, and immunohistochemical features of canine orbital hibernoma. *Veterinary Pathology* 51:563–568.

CASE 126

1 What is your interpretation? The cells seen in the picture are well-differentiated adipocytes. These cells are large, appear in groups or sometimes singly, and contain fat that stains negatively with Wright's, such that the cytoplasm appears clear. Nuclei are small, round, or ovoid and are frequently compressed and located to the periphery of the cell. These findings are supportive of lipoma, a benign tumor commonly observed in dogs and less frequently in cats. Surgical removal of lipomas may or may not be necessary. Surgical removal is recommended if there is associated pain, interference with local function, and/or predisposition to trauma. Infiltrative lipomas and their malignant counterpart liposarcomas are less common.

Editors' note: Sometimes, local fat will be aspirated and cannot be reliably differentiated from the adipose cells of a lipoma. If there is any doubt as to the presence of a discrete mass, surgical removal with histologic evaluation is recommended.

It is also important to remember that the presence of lipid material macroscopically is not sufficient for the diagnosis of a lipoma and this should be confirmed by the presence of adipose cells microscopically. There may be other lesions that contain a lipid component only because they are located close to or within the subcutaneous fat.

CASE 127

1 What is the structure shown? A ciliated protozoan organism. Note the cilia at each orifice and the esophagus and visible internal structure.

2 What is the significance of this finding? This is likely to be the result of fecal contamination.

3 What comments do you have regarding this finding? The organism is probably present due to poor preparation of the paracentesis site or contamination of the tube with fecal material or fecally contaminated water. The possibility of aspiration of gastrointestinal content is considered unlikely, since numerous bacteria (usually seen with gastrointestinal content aspiration) are not present in the background. A repeat collection should be considered, with attention to hygiene, collection site preparation, and specimen handling to prevent contamination.

CASE 128

1 Identify the components labeled 1, 2, 3, and 4 in the photomicrograph. These are the four most common components observed in this urine sediment sample: erythrocytes (1); leukocytes (2); bacteria, mostly rods and cocci in chains (3); and struvite crystals (4). In the dog, struvite crystals are commonly associated with bacterial infections. Note that at least 10^4 rods or 10^5 cocci/μl urine are required in order to be able to detect them on light microscopy.

2 What is your interpretation? The sediment is consistent with a urinary tract infection.

3 What is the most likely explanation for the positive reactive of the dipstick to nitrite and the presence of an alkaline pH? Two bacterial species (*Proteus* and *Enterococcus*) were detected by culture. *Proteus* is a bacterium able to reduce nitrate to nitrite and to produce urease. This enzyme cleaves urea in ammonia and carbon dioxide. Both compounds are responsible for the alkaline pH, which in turn favors the formation of struvite crystals.

CASE 129

1 **Describe the cytologic findings observed in photomicrograph 129a.** The smear is highly cellular and composed predominantly of poorly preserved neutrophils and low numbers of small lymphocytes, monocytes, and cells with pyknotic nuclei. A moderate amount of pink amorphous material is present in the hemodiluted background. Similar pink amorphous material and round to oval inclusions are also observed within neutrophils.

2 **How would you classify the joint disease?** Inflammatory joint disease.

3 **Name the cells labeled 1 and 2 in photomicrograph 129b, and explain their significance.** The cell labeled 1 is called a lupus erythematosus (LE) cell, and is a neutrophil containing intracytoplasmatic structures originating via opsonization by antinuclear antibodies. The presence of LE cells is highly suggestive of systemic lupus erythematosus (SLE). The cell labeled 2 is a ragocyte (neutrophil containing amorphous granular material); ragocytes are thought to represent neutrophils containing phagocytosed immune complexes or nuclear remnants and are commonly seen in association with immune-mediated polyarthropathies.

4 **What would be your main differential diagnosis?** Differential diagnoses for a nonerosive inflammatory arthropathy include infectious and immune-mediated causes. The most likely diagnosis in this case is an immune-mediated polyarthritis, as part of SLE.

SLE is a multisystem autoimmune disease, characterized by the formation of antibodies against a wide array of self-antigens and circulating immune complexes (type IV hypersensitivity reaction). These are formed and deposited in the glomerular basement membrane, synovial membrane, blood vessels, and skin, causing variable clinical signs according to the organ involved.

CASE 130

1 **What is the magenta substance visible in the background of the smear?** This is ultrasound gel, which is seen cytologically as a magenta-colored, granular precipitate in the background. This may occur diffusely or in focal areas on a slide. This is often an unwelcome artifact, as the gel can obscure cellular details and hamper the diagnostic process. It may also result in cell lysis or be confused with a necrotic background.

Further reading
Molyneux AJ, Coghill SB (1994) Cell lysis due to ultrasound gel in fine needle aspirates; an important new artefact in cytology. *Cytopathology* 5:41–45.

CASE 131
1 What type of fluid is present (fluid classification)? The elevated TP and NCC indicate an exudate.
2 What cells are present? The cells present are neutrophils (some immature) and macrophages. Although processed immediately, stain take up is very poor and, along with the physical parameters, this suggests an abdominal catastrophe such as intestinal torsion; however, microorganisms and plant material, which would indicate rupture of an intestinal viscus, are absent.
3 What is your interpretation? Peritonitis/possible torsion. Torsion was found on laparotomy.

CASE 132
1 Describe the cells shown in the smear. There is a clear background with a few erythrocytes and a cluster of cohesive basal-like epithelial cells. These have a small, round, relatively uniform nucleus, with granular chromatin and inconspicuous nucleoli. The cytoplasm is scant, basophilic, with indistinct cytoplasmic borders. Nuclei can be seen palisading along the edge (nuclei in a row) of the group in some areas.
2 What is your interpretation of these findings? The cytologic interpretation is of a cutaneous basilar epithelial neoplasm (previously called basal cell tumor or trichoblastoma). This general term is commonly used in cytopathology to identify a large group of usually benign skin neoplasms, frequently observed in domestic animals and arising from the epidermis, trichofollicular epithelium, or the adnexal structures. Subclassification of these neoplasms is not possible on cytopathology, and histopathology is recommended for further characterization.
3 What prognosis do you expect? Tumors in this group tend to be locally invasive but do not commonly metastasize. Therefore, if complete removal is achieved, the expected prognosis is good. Occasionally, there will be tumors with this morphology that exhibit more aggressive biological behavior.

CASE 133
1 Based on the cells present in photomicrograph 133a, what is the most likely cytologic diagnosis? The most likely diagnosis is a soft tissue sarcoma based on the groups of round to oval to spindle-shaped cells with indistinct cell margins. There are mildly increased numbers of neutrophils in the background, and occasional foamy macrophages containing debris. Thus, fibroplasia secondary to an inflammatory process is a consideration, but based on this image, the predominance of proliferating and atypical mesenchymal cells would be considered more consistent with neoplasia.

Answers

2 What are the four extremely large cells seen in photomicrograph 133b? How should these be interpreted? The four extremely large cells in **133b** are multinucleated giant cells, one of which can also be seen in the upper right corner of **133a**. While present in some sarcomas, these can also occur in inflammatory reactions, especially in response to foreign material or selected infectious agents such as *Mycobacterium*.

3 What etiology should be considered for the mass? This type of lesion in a cat may be associated with chronic inflammation or trauma, but a feline injection-site sarcoma should be considered. These tumors were previously referred to as vaccine-associated sarcomas; however, they have been renamed after discovering that other injectables can also cause this type of tumor, although the precise pathophysiologic mechanisms have not been elucidated. These tumors typically occur from 4 months to 3 years after injection, exhibiting local invasion, especially along fascial planes. Most are fibrosarcomas, although other sarcomas have been documented. Histologically, these tumors have a more significant inflammatory component than other sarcomas, which was noted in these cytology samples. Metastasis is more common, and was identified in this cat by imaging studies. The incidence of this form of sarcoma in the UK is much lower than documented in North America, possibly associated with different vaccine protocols. A genetic predisposition may play a role in which cats are affected.

CASE 134

1 What has caused the turquoise–blue, hazy appearance of the slide, and how can this be prevented? The submitted slide contains some erythrocytes. There are also some nucleated cells and a few bacteria that are suspected to be filamentous or in chains, but these are difficult or impossible to identify because of the poor cellular presentation and staining. This very blue staining with loss of cellular detail is caused by the slide coming into contact with formalin fumes before the staining process. Formalin is used as a fixative for histopathology samples; these fumes may fix the membranes of cells on cytology preparations, preventing the stain from entering the cell and staining it properly, with consequent loss of cellular detail. This can be prevented by ensuring that cytology smears are not exposed to formalin fumes in the area of collection, during transport, or in the area in which cytology specimens are handled prior to staining.

Editors' note: Cytology slides should always be packaged separately from histopathology specimens in order to avoid this contamination.

Answers

CASE 135

1 Describe the features seen in the photomicrographs. The photomicrographs show a background with many erythrocytes. There are moderate to many nucleated cells. These include a moderate number of neutrophils and a few macrophages, with an additional population of cells that occur singly and in cohesive groups. These cells show cytologic features of atypia. They have round to oval nuclei with clumped, dense chromatin and a single prominent nucleolus. The cytoplasm is moderate, with poorly distinct borders, occasionally showing cytoplasmic tails. The single cell shows distinct squamous differentiation with angular, crisply defined cytoplasmic borders.

2 What is your interpretation of this specimen? The cytologic features are consistent with an epithelial neoplasia, likely gastric squamous cell carcinoma.

3 What is the prognosis for this condition? The prognosis for gastric squamous cell carcinoma is poor. Its presence in abdominal fluid indicates that there has been rupture of the stomach wall or rupture of lymphatics containing malignant cells. These are the avenues of access into the abdominal fluid.

CASE 136

1 Describe the cells shown in the photomicrograph. The photomicrograph shows a main population of individual spindloid mesenchymal cells, rarely arranged in poorly cohesive groups and associated with amorphous eosinophilic material (matrix). These cells have moderate amounts of elongated lightly basophilic cytoplasm, with poorly distinct cytoplasmic borders. Nuclei are oval, with granular chromatin and indistinct round nucleoli. Anisocytosis and anisokaryosis are moderate. A few blood-derived neutrophils are also noted.

2 What are your differential diagnoses based on these cytologic findings? These cytologic findings are supportive of a mesenchymal proliferation. Differential diagnoses include reactive fibroplasia or mesenchymal neoplasia, of which fibroma, well-differentiated fibrosarcoma, or sarcoid are the primary considerations. It is not possible to distinguish among these possibilities based on the histologic features alone, but the histologic findings confirmed sarcoid. The characteristic arrangement of spindloid cells perpendicular to the epithelial basement membrane typical of sarcoid was present.

Sarcoid represents the most common mesenchymal skin tumor in the equine species. It appears as a single (occasionally multiple) skin lesion; preferred locations include head, neck, extremities, and ventrum. Bovine papillomavirus types 1 and 2 are causally associated with the development and pathogenesis of equine sarcoids, although infection alone is not sufficient for tumor production. A breed predisposition (e.g. Quarter Horses, Arabians, and Appaloosas) is considered likely.

Answers

CASE 137

1 What is the structure shown? A Curschmann's spiral. It has a dense, central, twisted core, surrounded by a lighter mantle of less dense mucus.

2 What is the significance of this finding in a respiratory cytology specimen? Curschmann's spirals are a reflection of mucostasis. One end of a strand of mucus is fixed within the airway and the other end is 'free', allowing twisting of the core and accumulation of the less dense mantle of mucus with time. Curschmann's spirals are a nonspecific finding, but they may occur in any condition where there is static mucus. They may contribute to airway narrowing and 'functional' obstruction of airways.

CASE 138

1 Identify the cell population present in the photomicrograph, and describe the most relevant cytologic findings. The samples are good in quality and cellularity; there is a main population of nucleated cells, mostly naked nuclei on a slightly basophilic and granular background. These occasionally form small aggregates, showing a pseudoacinar arrangement or forming nests and ribbon-like aggregates. Intact cells have a round/oval shape, a high N:C ratio, and small to moderate amounts of granular basophilic cytoplasm; nuclei are round to oval, with a reticular, coarse or finely stippled chromatin and indistinct nucleoli. Cellular atypia is slight.

2 What is your interpretation of these findings? These cytologic features are primarily suggestive of a neuroendocrine tumor, likely pheochromocytoma, and are supported by the location of the mass. Differential diagnoses may include an adrenocortical tumor and an adrenal metastasis from another malignant neuroendocrine neoplasia. The former is considered unlikely, since neoplastic cells in adrenocortical neoplasms commonly have a low N:C ratio and large amounts of basophilic, vacuolated cytoplasm. Metastases of other neuroendocrine neoplasms to the adrenal gland also are rare.

3 What additional tests could be used to support and confirm the diagnosis? Measurement of catecholamine metabolites in urine and plasma is now considered a good screening test to support the diagnosis of pheochromocytoma and to rule out a neoplasia of adrenocortical origin. However, these metabolites are unstable, they require special sample handling, and can be measured only by a limited number of laboratories. Definitive diagnosis requires histopathology and immunohistochemistry.

Further reading

Bertazzolo W, Didier M, Gelain ME et al. (2014) Accuracy of cytology in distinguishing adrenocortical tumors from pheochromocytoma in companion animals. *Veterinary Clinical Pathology* 43:453–459.

Gostelow R, Bridger N, Syme HM (2013) Plasma-free metanephrine and free normetanephrine measurement for the diagnosis of pheochromocytoma in dogs. *Journal of Veterinary Internal Medicine* 27:83–90.

CASE 139

1 Describe the features shown in the smear. There are a few vacuolated columnar epithelial cells with a few nuclei that have been stripped of cytoplasm. There is a moderate number of neutrophils and a few macrophages. Within some of the macrophages, and free in the background of the smear, are numerous small, oval organisms that stain red–orange and are consistent with yeasts. These are smaller than erythrocytes and do not contain homogeneous hemoglobin within the cell membrane.

2 What is your interpretation of these findings? The cytologic findings are consistent with uterine yeast infection.

Editors' note: Equine uterine fungal infections may present with either yeast or hyphae. It is very uncommon to see both forms in one animal, since the individual uterine environment is usually only suitable for one type or the other.

CASE 140

1 Describe the features seen. Many columnar epithelial cells with oval, basal nuclei containing finely stippled chromatin can be seen. The cytoplasm is columnar and finely vacuolated. A few small lymphocytes are seen in the background. No neutrophils or infectious agents are visible.

2 What is your interpretation of these findings? The cytologic features are consistent with normal reproductive status and active cycling.

3 Why is this important? It is important to know this since the cytology indicates that this mare is ready to breed and does not need any treatment prior to breeding. It is important to compare the results of uterine cytology with that of bacterial culture (often required by breeding farms upon entry). In this mare there was a scant growth of *Streptococcus* species obtained on culture, but the cytology indicates that this is likely to be a false-positive result since inflammation is not present. Correlation of the uterine cytology and culture is needed to determine if inflammation is present in the face of a positive culture. If so, treatment is indicated. If not, treatment is not indicated.

Further reading
Freeman KP, Roszel JF, Slusher SH (1986) Patterns in equine endometrial cytologic smears. *Compendium on Continuing Education for the Practicing Veterinarian* 8(7): 349–360.
Slusher SH, Freeman KP, Roszel JF (1985) Infertility diagnosis in mares using endometrial biopsy, culture and aspirate cytology. *Proceedings of the 31st Convention of the American Association of Equine Practitioners*, Toronto, p. 165.

CASE 141

1 Describe the cytologic findings, and give your cytologic interpretation. The sample is highly cellular and is characterized by clusters of cohesive epithelial cells. These are occasionally arranged in tubules and rosettes or acini. The cells are medium sized with indistinct cytoplasmic borders, pale blue cytoplasm, a high N:C ratio, and a round to oval nucleus. Eosinophilic amorphous material (likely secretion) is occasionally seen within these rosettes. Mild cellular pleomorphism is observed. These cytologic features are supportive of an anal sac adenocarcinoma.

2 What additional tests would you recommend? Evaluation of total and/or ionized calcium is recommended since paraneoplastic hypercalcemia is observed in more than 25% of the dogs affected by this neoplasia. Abdominal ultrasound of iliac lymph nodes is strongly encouraged, since this is a very common site of metastasis for this malignant and invasive neoplasia. This will also help for clinical staging and prognostic purposes.

Editors' note: The causes of hypercalcemia of malignancy vary and include ectopic production of parathyroid hormone or parathyroid-related peptide by the neoplasia and extensive lytic bone metastases.

CASE 142

1 Describe the findings in the smear. There is a moderate number of erythrocytes, in clumps, and frequent spermatozoa in the background. The spermatozoa have pale blue heads and pale gray tails, some of which are curled or have been detached. No neutrophils or infectious agents are visible.

2 What is the significance of these findings? The spermatozoa are an incidental finding in a prostatic washing since there is usually ejaculation when the reproductive/urinary system is massaged prior to collection. The erythrocytes confirm the presence of blood, but no inflammation is seen.

No transitional epithelial cells are seen in this smear. They are often present in prostatic washings. In this case they were represented in other fields and did not have features consistent with malignancy. Sometimes, transitional cell carcinoma will occur in the prostatic urethra and grow or expand into the prostate gland. Therefore, evaluation of a prostatic washing is valuable because transitional epithelial cells from the prostatic urethra are usually represented.

3 What other recommendations might you have? Since no columnar epithelial cells consistent with prostatic gland origin are seen, this precludes evaluation for features of hyperplasia or malignancy. If additional evaluation of the prostate gland is desired, ultrasound-guided fine needle aspiration of the prostate gland is recommended. This technique has a high probability of obtaining a representative specimen since it samples from the prostate gland directly. Ultrasound-guided

FNAs of the prostate gland have replaced prostatic washings as the preferred specimen of choice for evaluation of suspected prostatic abnormalities and, since ultrasound is widely available, they are frequently submitted to the laboratory. Iatrogenic tumor seeding after cytologic and/or histologic biopsies is a rare event and has been reported in the literature.

Further reading
Teske E (2009) Urogenital cytology. *Presented at the 34th World Small Animal Veterinary Congress WSAVA 2009*, São Paulo, Brazil.

CASE 143

1 What is the cytologic interpretation of this CSF? There is a markedly increased number of inflammatory cells present in the slide (pleocytosis). These cells predominantly consist of nondegenerate neutrophils (>80%), with small numbers of mononuclear cells, mostly macrophages. No bacterial or other infectious agents are seen.

2 What are the possible differential diagnoses? Neutrophilic pleocytosis can be associated with infectious or noninfectious causes including bacterial or fungal meningoencephalitis, steroid-responsive meningitis–arteritis (SRMA), and underlying neoplasia. Less common causes include post myelography reactions or trauma. These cytologic findings and results of body fluid analysis, together with the clinical history (neck pain, pyrexia) and the nondegenerate appearance of the neutrophils, are highly suggestive of SRMA. Visualization of bacteria in CSF is frequently not possible, even in confirmed cases of bacterial meningoencephalitis, therefore bacterial culture of the CSF sample is recommended to help exclude a bacterial etiology.

CASE 144

1 What is the elongated, brown, segmented structure in the lower right/central portion of the smear? A fungal spore of the genus *Alternaria*.

2 What is the significance of this finding? When present in small numbers these are considered to be an insignificant finding and should not be interpreted as evidence of fungal infection. When present in moderate to large numbers they may indicate an increased environmental load and/or decreased pulmonary clearance of environmental spores. Correlation with the spore and pollen count, evaluation to determine if moldy hay may be present, and consideration of environmental factors and other evidence of pulmonary disease may be needed to determine their significance when present in moderate to large numbers. Often they are accompanied by other types of spores and sometimes with pigmented fungal hyphal fragments.

Answers

CASE 145

1 Describe the cytologic findings seen in the photomicrographs, and give your interpretation. The two photomicrographs represent different areas of the same preparation. The background is lightly basophilic (proteinaceous) and contains a small amount of blood. There are numerous anucleated squamous epithelial cells (squames), often in groups. They consist of polygonal and flattened anucleated cells, which are often folded. They are characterized by well-defined cell borders and a dense, lightly to moderately basophilic cytoplasm. These findings are consistent with an epidermal or follicular inclusion cyst. Epidermal inclusion cysts are non-neoplastic skin lesions that more frequently occur in older dogs. These may form as a result of traumatic embedding of epidermal fragments or a congenital anomaly of epidermal development. In cases of rupture of the cystic wall, the exposure of the keratin to the surrounding tissue can elicit an endogenous foreign body reaction characterized by purulent to pyogranulomatous inflammation. In these cases, the inflammatory cells are often found surrounding the squames, as seen in photomicrograph **145b**. The prognosis is excellent and surgical excision is curative.

2 What are the structures pointed to by the arrows in 145a. What is the significance of these structures? The polygonal and negatively staining structures indicated by the arrows are cholesterol crystals. They derive from the cellular membrane lipid and indicate cell degeneration and/or static secretion. They are often seen in epidermal inclusion cysts and may also be found in chronic/resolving hematomas.

Editors' note: Sometimes, tumors of epithelial origin may contain cysts with the same contents as illustrated in this case. Therefore, surgical removal is always recommended, with histologic evaluation to determine if there may be adjacent neoplasia that is not represented in the sample.

Further reading
Gross TL, Ihrke PJ, Walder EJ *et al.* (2005) *Skin Disease of the Dog and Cat: Clinical and Histopathologic Diagnosis*, 2nd edn. Wiley-Blackwell, Ames, pp. 604–640.

CASE 146

1 What kind of crystals are shown on the photomicrograph? Struvite (magnesium-ammonium-phosphate), which is the most common crystal found in the urine sediment of cats.

2 What do they tell you from a clinical point of view with regard to the other findings? The presence of struvite crystals in this cat's urine sediment indicates that there is supersaturation of the components of the crystals (Mg, NH_3, and phosphate). This is the precondition for the formation of these crystals. The crystals on the photomicrograph are beginning to dissolve, indicating an aging sample.

There were no clinical signs reported. The blood results support slight dehydration with an increase in TP and albumin; the USG is normal–high and the pH is in the alkaline range, favoring the formation of struvite crystals. However, *in-vitro* formation of these crystals cannot be entirely excluded since the sample was not examined immediately following collection.

The strongly positive WBC reaction on the dipstick is frequently a spurious reaction in cat's urine and must be disregarded. Unlike in dogs, the formation of struvite crystals in cats is not associated with urinary tract infection.

In conclusion, the finding of struvite crystals has to be interpreted with care in cats without clinical signs, especially in voided samples that are not examined immediately after collection.

Further reading
Osborne CA, Lulich JP, Polzin DJ *et al.* (1999) Medical dissolution and prevention of canine struvite urolithiasis. Twenty years of experience. *Veterinary Clinics of North America: Small Animal Practice* **29**:73–111.

CASE 147

1 Classify the pleural fluid. An exudate. The TP is >30g/l and the NCC is >5 × 10^9/l.
2 Based on the macroscopic (147a) and microscopic (147b, c) appearance of the pleural fluid, what further laboratory tests would you like to request? Fluid cholesterol and triglyceride concentrations.
3 Given the results of the tests requested above, how would you now reclassify this fluid? Chylous effusion. This interpretation is based on a fluid cholesterol: triglyceride ratio of <1.
4 List the most common causes of chylous effusions in cats. Chylous effusions form when there is a physical (e.g. mediastinal mass) or functional (cardiovascular disease) obstruction of lymphatics, resulting in increased pressure (lymphangiectasia) and, less commonly, rupture of the thoracic duct (trauma). In cats, cardiomyopathy is a common cause.

Editors' note: Identification of chylous fluid in a body cavity is consistent with lymph stasis. The body fluid analysis may reflect a modified transudate or exudate. The macroscopic milky appearance and presence of chylomicrons and lipid droplets cytologically may vary, depending on metabolic status and how recently a fatty meal has been consumed. Chylous effusions contain higher triglyceride levels compared with serum, which has a fluid:serum triglyceride ratio usually >3:1. In addition, a fluid cholesterol:triglyceride ratio of <1 was proposed to be characteristic of a chylous effusion.

Answers

A variety of conditions and disease processes may result in chylous effusions, as noted above. In addition to cardiac insufficiency, the presence of a mass (abscess, hematoma, granuloma, or tumor) interfering with vascular/lymphatic return, and rupture of the thoracic duct, chylous effusions have been reported with diaphragmatic hernia, lung torsion, chronic coughing, chronic vomiting, steatitis, biliary cirrhosis, congenital lymphatic abnormalities, lymphangiectasia, and as an idiopathic condition.

Further reading
Baker R, Lumsden JH (2000) *Color Atlas of Cytology of the Dog and Cat*, 1st edn. Mosby, St. Louis, pp. 23–29.
Meadows RL, MacWilliams PS (1994) Chylous effusions revisited. *Veterinary Clinical Pathology* **23**(2):54–62.

CASE 148
1 What cells are present? The cells vary widely in size but are distinctly spindle shaped. They have tails of basophilic cytoplasm and oval nuclei with clumped chromatin. There is a lot of cell debris, suggesting cell fragility and necrosis.
2 What is the cytologic interpretation? The presence of clusters of spindle-shaped cells alien to this location indicates a spindle cell tumor/sarcoma is likely. A diagnosis of rhabdomyosarcoma was made on histopathologic examination.

Editors' note: Diagnosis of 'likely sarcoma', as mentioned in the discussion of other cases in this book, may be as specific a diagnosis as can be made based on routine cytologic evaluation. In some cases of rhabdomyosarcoma there may be sufficient organization of intracytoplasmic filaments to demonstrate cross striations typical of skeletal muscle. This is usually only present in a few cells, if any. Immunohistochemical demonstration of actin muscle and desmin in the cells with malignant features is supportive of muscle origin, while demonstration of actin sarcomeric and myglobin is considered specific for striated muscle origin.

CASE 149
1 Identify the organism. *Prototheca* spp. Protothecosis is cause by the achlorophylic algae *Prototheca*. Infection is through sewage contaminated aquatic environmental sources. Only two of the three species of *Prototheca*, *Prototheca zophii* and *Prototheca wickerhamii*, are pathogenic. *P. zophii* is the most frequent isolate in dogs with disseminated disease, while *P. wicherhamii* is associated with dermal lesions. In cytologic preparations, the organism is approximately 4 microns by 10 microns, round to oval, and occasionally reniform, with a thin refractile wall and basophilic granular

internal structures. The typical internal septation that forms during endosporulation and is seen in histologic sections is not as easily appreciated, if at all, in cytologic preparations.

Further reading
Rizzi TE, Cowell RL, Meinkoth JH *et al*. (2006) Subretinal aspirate from a dog. *Veterinary Clinical Pathology* 35:111–113.

CASE 150

1 Describe the features seen in the smears. There is a basophilic proteinaceous background with large clear lipid vacuoles and nucleated cells, either individual or arranged in groups. These are large, with round to oval nuclei, granular chromatin, and often with a single prominent nucleolus. The cytoplasm is moderate and often contains one or several crisply defined clear vacuoles.
2 What is your cytologic interpretation? Mesenchymal proliferation, likely neoplastic. The lipid vacuoles and the vacuolated cytoplasm are highly suggestive of liposarcoma.
3 Are there any confirmatory tests that can/should be done? Sudan III staining of an unfixed, air-dried smear would be able to confirm the presence of lipid. The Sudan III stains lipid red to pink. Oil Red O stain can also be used.

Further reading
Masserdotti C, Bonfanti U, De Lorenzi D *et al*. (2006). Use of Oil Red O stain in the cytologic diagnosis of canine liposarcoma. *Veterinary Clinical Pathology* 35(1):37–41.

CASE 151

1 Describe the cytologic findings, and give your cytologic interpretation. The smears contains variable numbers of hepatocytes with abundant foamy cytoplasm, distended by small, variably sized, clear globules, frequently obscuring the nuclear outline, overall indicative of microvesicular steatosis. Similar globules are also dispersed in the background.
2 What are the most frequent causes of this condition? Microvesicular steatosis is commonly observed secondary to severe hypoxia, intoxication, adverse drug reactions, or an imbalance of lipoprotein excretion. In contrast, macrovesicular steatosis (characterized by the presence of large clear intracytoplasmic vacuoles displacing the nucleus to the periphery) – also known as hepatic lipidosis – occurs most frequently as a consequence of prolonged starvation and/or metabolic diseases, including diabetes mellitus. The cytologic features of these two conditions can sometimes overlap and distinction on cytology is not always possible. Chronic kidney disease with severe nonregenerative anemia was confirmed in this cat.

CASE 152

1 Describe the cells shown in the images. In a proteinaceous and mildly hemodiluted background, there are 'spindle cells' in small aggregates or individually. The cells are mononucleated with occasional multinucleated forms. They display moderate anisokaryosis and anisocytosis. The nuclei are medium-large, oval and contain granular chromatin. Occasionally, 1–2 small and round nucleoli are observed. The cytoplasm is lightly basophilic with poorly defined contours, and often contains sparse small, clear, punctate vacuoles.

2 What is your interpretation and recommendation? In this particular case, providing a definitive diagnosis is very challenging and the main differential diagnoses are a relapse of the previous sarcoma and a reactive fibroplasia due to scar tissue formation secondary to the surgery. The radiotherapy course is an additional confounding factor, as this often causes damage to the tissue cells, leading to cellular dysplasia. In this situation, the cytologist can only provide a subjective interpretation, but histopathology is ultimately suggested to confirm the diagnosis.

Editors' note: The limitation of cytology in differentiating malignant mesenchymal tumors from benign proliferations is well known and is mainly due to the inability to evaluate the mitotic activity of the cell proliferation, the encapsulation and infiltration of the mass, and some architectural features. The presence or absence of inflammation in the lesion may not be of any aid, as sarcomas are often associated with a secondary inflammation; on the other hand, reactive and inflammatory processes can cause cellular dysplasia. In spite of these limitations, cytology remains a helpful tool in the diagnosis of mesenchymal tumors and helps in excluding other diseases such as other kinds of tumors and inflammation.

Further reading
DeMay R (2012) *The Art and Science of Cytopathology*, 2nd edn. ASCP Press, Chicago, pp. 635–749.

CASE 153

1 Describe the features shown. There is a mucoid background with a few neutrophils and erythrocytes. There is some refractile crystalline debris and several intertwined fungal hyphae. The hyphae are narrow (several microns in diameter) and irregularly septate. No branching is illustrated in these fragments, but in other fields the hyphae exhibited dichotomous branching.

2 What is your interpretation of these findings? The features are consistent with active (neutrophilic) inflammation and the presence of fungal hyphae is suggestive of nasal aspergillosis.

3 What additional tests might be recommended? A fungal culture with evaluation of reproductive structures is needed for a definitive diagnosis of aspergillosis. Correlation with an *Aspergillus* antibody titer may be helpful in documenting exposure and an immune response to this organism. However, false-positive results may occur when there has been exposure but no current infection, and false-negative results may occur, particularly with early infection or infection in an immunocompromised animal that may not be capable of mounting an immune response. Correlation with the endoscopic appearance also may be helpful if white plaque-like lesions composed of fungal hyphae can be seen.

CASE 154

1 What cells are represented in 154a? The cells shown here are sebaceous epithelial cells (sebocytes). They are well differentiated and are characterized by a small, round and condensed nucleus and abundant, heavily vacuolated cytoplasm. The vacuoles are generally small, clear and discrete.

2 What is your diagnosis? These cytologic findings indicate either a sebaceous adenoma or hyperplasia. These two forms cannot be distinguished on cytology but have the same benign clinical behavior. Identical lesions found on the eyelid margins are called meibomian gland adenomas and arise from specialized tarsal sebaceous glands.

Sebaceous adenomas most frequently occur in older dogs and can be solitary or multiple and often alopecic. The prognosis is excellent and surgical excision is curative.

3 What are the cells indicated by the arrows in 154b. What is the significance of these cells? The cells pointed to by the arrows are cuboidal reserve epithelial cells. They are normally present in low numbers in sebaceous adenomas. The presence of high numbers of reserve epithelial cells, especially if they exceed the mature sebocytes, is supportive of a sebaceous epithelioma. Historically, the WHO classified sebaceous epitheliomas as low-grade carcinomas, although these tumors often behave in a benign fashion.

CASE 155

1 What cell types are present in the photomicrograph? There is a clear background with small numbers of RBCs. Most of the nucleated cells present are small lymphocytes (1). There are also small numbers of medium and large lymphoid cells (2). Large individual cells with a round to oval nucleus and wispy pale blue cytoplasm are also present in low numbers (3).

2 What is your interpretation? Thymoma. The large mononuclear cells with poorly defined cytoplasmic borders are thymic epithelial cells. These can occur singly, as seen in this photomicrograph, or in clusters, and commonly lack criteria of malignancy.

Thymoma is a neoplasm originating from the epithelial cells of the thymus, which are admixed with non-neoplastic lymphoid cells, mainly small lymphocytes. Low numbers of mast cells may also be observed in cytologic preparations from thymomas and may help in reaching a final diagnosis, especially when cytologic samples lack the high level of cellularity that is usually needed for a confident diagnosis and lack epithelial cells. Histopathologic examination is recommended when a definitive diagnosis is not possible on the sole basis of cytology. Flow cytometry analysis is the preferred method for identification of thymoma, although PARR testing may also be considered. In thymomas, the lymphoid component is expected to be polyclonal and composed of >10% of lymphocytes co-expressing CD4 and CD8, whereas lymphomas are characterized by a monoclonal population of lymphoid cells, most commonly T cell in origin.

Further reading
Lana S, Plaza S, Hampe K *et al.* (2006) Diagnosis of mediastinal masses in dogs by flow cytometry. *Journal of Veterinary Internal Medicine* **20:**1161–1165.

CASE 156
1 What is the cytologic interpretation of this CSF. There is a markedly increased number of inflammatory cells (pleocytosis). These cells consist of a mixture of nondegenerate neutrophils (60–70%) and large mononuclear cells, likely macrophages (30–40%). No bacteria or other infectious agents can be seen. The cytologic interpretation is a mixed pleocytosis.

2 What are the possible differential diagnoses? Mixed cell pleocytosis can be seen with a wide variety of pathologic conditions including steroid-responsive meningitis–arteritis (SRMA), meningoencephalitis of unknown origin (MEUO), protozoal disease (e.g. *Toxoplasma* or *Neospora*), fungal infections (*Cryptococcus*), viral infection (*Distemper*), or underlying neoplasia.

In this case, bacterial culture was negative and the dog was treated with immunosuppressive medication and recovered well, suggesting an immune-mediated etiology (either SRMA or MEUO).

CASE 157
1 What cells are present in the center of the photomicrograph (arrow)? There is a macrophage surrounded by erythroid precursors, mainly metarubricytes and rubricytes. This arrangement is referred to as an 'erythroblastic island'.

2 What process does this represent, and when does it occur? Erythroid precursors are commonly observed in the spleen as part of the process of extramedullary hematopoiesis (EMH). Myeloid precursors and megakaryocytes are also usually noted. Pronounced EMH, particularly of the erythroid lineage, usually occurs in response to acute or chronic anemia, but may also noted with myeloproliferative disorders and lymphoma. An erythroblastic island is a hematopoietic niche, with the macrophage providing iron for the developing erythroid cells and phagocytosing the extruded nuclei as the red cells mature.

Further reading
Chasis JA, Mohandas N (2008) Erythroblastic islands: niches for erythropoiesis. *Blood* 112:470–478.

CASE 158

1 Describe the findings seen in the photomicrographs. The aspirate is characterized by low numbers of macrophages found individually or, more frequently, in small clusters. These have a large amount of pale basophilic cytoplasm that consistently contains numerous elongated, opaque basophilic structures of phagocytosed material (1). Similar structures are also found extracellularly, in close proximity to the inflammatory cells. Low numbers of multinucleated giant cells (2) are also observed. Occasional hematoidin crystals (3) are present, supportive of a low-grade chronic hemorrhage.

2 What is your interpretation? Gossypiboma. This is a granulomatous inflammatory lesion that forms secondary to a retained surgical sponge/swab. The elongated structures that are seen extracellularly and within macrophages are consistent with the fibers from the surgical sponge. These synthetic fibers are difficult or impossible to degrade, and the body responds to their presence by encapsulating and walling off the foreign material and forming a sterile granuloma. In this case, a retained surgical swab was found at surgery, confirming the cytologic diagnosis of a gossypiboma (158c).

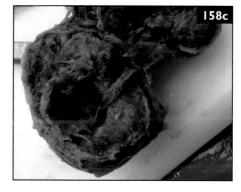

Further reading
Putwain S, Archer J (2009) What is your diagnosis? Intra-abdominal mass aspirate from a spayed dog with abdominal pain. *Veterinary Clinical Pathology* 38:253–256.

Answers

CASE 159

1 Which interpretation best describes this smear: (a) normal; (b) reactive/ hyperplastic; (c) metastatic tumor; or (d) multiple myeloma? (b). Hyperplastic/ reactive lymph nodes are enlarged on clinical palpation and aspirates are usually highly cellular. Small lymphocytes predominate but there is an increase of the medium and large forms, which account for more that 15% of the entire lymphoid population. Increased numbers of plasma cells (marked *) may also be observed. Occasional Mott and tingible body macrophages may also be seen.

2 What are Mott cells (see inset) and tingible body macrophages? Mott cells are plasma cells with basophilic cytoplasm and contain clear vacuoles, called Russell bodies. The nature of Russell bodies is debatable but some authors suggest that they represent accumulations of immunoglobulins (Ig) within vesicles. The proposed underlying mechanism is a defect (partial or complete) in secretion of Ig. Tingible body macrophages are macrophages that contain phagocytosed remnants of cellular material. Increased numbers are seen with increased apoptosis/ 'cytorrhexis' and are common in lymphoproliferative disorders.

3 List the differentials for reactive/hyperplastic lymph nodes. This process may be observed in any local or generalized antigenic response, and may include infection, inflammation, immune-mediated processes, and neoplasia. Specific infectious conditions that may induce lymphoid hyperplasia include ehrlichiosis, FIV/FeLV infection, Rocky Mountain spotted fever, and Lyme's disease.

Editors' note: Tick-borne diseases are important differential diagnoses when lymphoid hyperplasia is observed cytologically. Other conditions that commonly result in generalized lymphoid hyperplasia include diffuse skin disease, external parasitism, fungal disease, and systemic infection/sepsis. Generalized or regional lymph node enlargement with a cytologic interpretation of lymphoid hyperplasia may occur with tumor or localized irritation or injury. Idiopathic enlargement of lymph nodes may also occur, and lymph node enlargement in young animals may occur as new antigens are encountered. In the absence of a specific cause for lymphoid stimulation recognizable in cytologic preparations, continued investigation for an underlying cause is recommended.

Further reading

Hsu SM, Hso PL, McMillan PN *et al.* (1982) Russell bodies: a light and electron microscopic immunoperoxidase study. *American Journal of Clinical Pathology* 77:26–31.

Valenciano AC, Cowell RL (2014) (eds) *Cowell and Tyler's Diagnostic Cytology and Hematology of the Dog and Cat*, 4th edn. Mosby/Elsevier, St. Louis, pp. 185–186.

CASE 160
1 Describe the cells and the background material present in the photomicrographs. Round to oval to polyhedral to stellate cells occur individually or loosely aggregated in a bright pink granular matrix. The cells are characterized by moderate to abundant amounts of pale blue cytoplasm. Each cell contains a single round to oval to angular nucleus. Occasional binucleated cells are observed. There are also variably sized, well-defined clear vacuoles in the background most consistent with lipid.

2 What is the most likely cytologic diagnosis? The most likely cytologic diagnosis is chondrosarcoma, which was confirmed histologically after complete surgical excision of the lesion. The presence of abundant and deeply eosinophilic matrix filling the background is common in bone tumors and is considered characteristic for chondroma/chondrosarcoma. However, cytologic differentiation of bone tumors is not always possible, and histopathology is needed for a definitive diagnosis.

CASE 161
1 Describe the findings seen in the photomicrograph. The photomicrograph shows variable numbers of well-differentiated hepatocytes, occasionally with rarefacted clear cytoplasm and frequently containing small amounts of intracytoplasmic green pigment. There are also variable numbers of segmented neutrophils, frequently associated with the hepatocytes and occasionally forming small groups (indicated by the arrow).

2 What is your interpretation based on these cytologic findings? These findings are indicative of a neutrophilic inflammation (hepatitis/cholangitis).

Editors' note: The significance of neutrophils in cytologic samples from most organs is frequently difficult to interpret, since it may be spurious due to hemodilution. A truly neutrophilic inflammation is suggested when a high concentration of neutrophils is observed relative to the erythrocytes and/or when neutrophils are intimately associated with or within the hepatocyte clumps. Histopathology is recommended to confirm these findings and to differentiate between primary parenchymal inflammatory processes (hepatitis) versus inflammation of the biliary tract (cholangitis).

CASE 162
1 Describe the features observed in the photomicrographs, and provide a general description. The samples are highly cellular with good preservation. A monomorphic population of round to polygonal or elongated cells is seen throughout the smear.

These cells are mostly individual and occasionally form small groups, showing a perivascular arrangement. The latter is characterized by central capillary spaces surrounded by clustered interstitial cells. Cells have variable N:C ratios, with moderate to abundant pink to pale purple cytoplasm with distinct borders; sparse to moderate, small, punctate, uniform intracytoplasmic vacuoles are also noted, together with rare dark blue to black cytoplasmic granules (162a). Nuclei are round to oval, central to paracentral, with variably coarsely clumped chromatin and a single small, relatively inconspicuous round nucleolus. Anisocytosis and anisokaryosis are mild to moderate.

2 **What is your interpretation?** Interstitial cell tumor (Leydig cell tumor). These are common testicular neoplasms in the dog, although they only rarely cause testicular enlargement and, therefore, are infrequently aspirated for cytology analysis. They are associated with testosterone production, and may contribute to the development of prostatic diseases and perianal gland neoplasms.

CASE 163

1 **What is the likely origin of these cells?** The submitted sample harvested a few small groups of well-differentiated mesothelial cells. Note the 'slits' or 'windows' between individual cells, indicative of a lack of tight intercellular junctions between the cells, in the lower left portion of the photomicrograph; these slits or windows support a mesothelial origin rather than epithelial cells, between which tight junctions occur. These cells do not display any cytologic features of atypia, and only occasionally contain a pink, round intracytoplasmic inclusion. These can occasionally be observed within mesothelial cells and have an unknown clinical significance. The presence of mesothelial cells is a common finding in aspirates from internal organs and likely reflects accidental traumatic exfoliation of the serous membrane covering the abdominal cavity.

Further reading
Koss LG, Melamed MR *(2005) Koss' Diagnostic Cytology and Its Histopathologic Bases*, 5th edn. Lippincott Williams and Wilkins, Philadelphia, p. 925.

CASE 164

1 **Describe the cytologic findings observed in the photomicrograph.** A population of round cells is observed in a clear background with small numbers of RBCs. These nucleated cells have moderate amounts of clear to pale blue cytoplasm, occasionally containing a few purple (magenta) granules. Nuclei are eccentrically placed, round to oval, with a finely stippled chromatin pattern and some nuclei contain indistinct, small round nucleoli. Anisocytosis and anisokaryosis are mild.

These findings are supportive of poorly granulated mast cells. Two eosinophils are also present on the upper right and right center of the image. A small amount of dense, pink, amorphous material is observed on the left center of the picture and is consistent with degraded collagen.

2 What is your interpretation? Mast cell tumor (MCT), poorly granulated.

Editors' note: The mast cells in this case have only a few intracytoplasmic purple granules. This lack of granulation may sometimes be an obstacle to achieving a definitive diagnosis of MCT. Detailed scanning of the smear at high-power field (×100) may help to identify granules when present in low numbers. The concurrent presence of eosinophils, fibroblasts, and collagenolysis further support this. If needed, special cyto/histochemical stains (e.g. Toloudine Blue) may be performed to identify these granules. Diff-Quik® may also not stain MCT granules well and, when this occurs, may result in difficulty in determining the correct diagnosis or attributing a poorer grade to the tumor.

The lack of granulation, especially when associated with other cytologic features of malignancy (e.g. marked anisocytosis, anisokaryosis, prominent nucleoli, and presence of atypical mitotic figures), suggests the presence of a more aggressive, high-grade MCT. However, histopathology examination remains the gold standard for tumor grading.

CASE 165

1 Describe the features shown in the photomicrograph. There is a basophilic and vacuolated background with areas of necrosis and fibrillary pink strands. Intact monolayers of cells comprise mainly intermediate lymphoid cells with slightly irregular, often extended, light blue cytoplasm that typically has variably distinct, irregularly distributed to focal azurophilic granulation. Their nuclei are roughly circular with irregularly clumped chromatin. Two mitotic figures (top center and lower right) are also seen in this view.

2 What is your interpretation of these findings? Cutaneous lymphoma. PCR clonality testing on the smears, or fresh aspirates for flow cytometry immunophenotyping, is required for further characterization of the cells if histopathology and immunohistochemistry are not used. Staging investigations, including hematology, biochemistry, and diagnostic imaging, also are recommended.

CASE 166

1 What are the organisms shown in the photomicrographs? The organisms are consistent with *Dermatophilus congolensis*. *Dermatophilus* is a gram-positive bacterium belonging to the class Actinobacteria. It is the causative agent of dermatophilosis, also know as mud fever or rain-scab in horses. *Dermatophilus* can also affect cattle, sheep, humans, and other species and is widespread in tropical regions. In cattle it is usually known as cutaneous streptotrichosis.

Dermatophilus is infrequently found in moderate climates. In horses, two clinical entities have been described: a winter and a summer form. The winter form tends to be more severe in clinical course and is typically associated with the scabs seen in the case described here.

2 How are they identified? Only a few organisms may be seen during cytologic examination of the scabs in chronic cases. Therefore, an adequate number of slides should be prepared and examined. The organisms are seen in the photomicrograph **166b** (unstained sample, ×100, oil) as branching (pseudo-) hyphae of about 1 μm in diameter, consisting of 2–6 parallel rows of coccoid endospores in pairs, resembling railroad tracks or stacked coins. Definitive diagnosis can be made by bacterial culture on blood agar under microaerophilic conditions. The photomicrograph **166c** shows a smear made from material of cultured *Dermatophilus congolensis*. For large scale serologic and epidemiologic surveys, indirect fluorescent antibody technique, ELISA, and PCR assays are available.

3 What are the differentials? Differentials include dermatophytosis and immune-mediated scaling diseases (e.g. pemphigus foliaceous).

Further reading
Szczepanik M, Golynski M, Pomorska D *et al.* (2006) Dermatophilosis in a horse – a case report. *Bulletin of the Veterinary Institute in Pulawy* **50**:619–622.

Frequently asked questions

FAQ1 How can cytology be of value to me in practice?

Cytology can be of value in determining a diagnosis, a type of process, and/or possible differential diagnoses. It may be of benefit for prognosis, treatment planning (including surgical or medical approach), and client education. It may also be of benefit for monitoring the progression of conditions or determining response to treatment.

When the use of cytology is being contemplated, the following should be considered:

- The value of cytology lies in its ability to affect the progress or handling of a case in a manner that would not have been possible had cytology not been done.
- If the use of cytology does not have the potential to affect your approach or handling of a case, its use is questionable.
- If cytology does not consistently provide a high degree of useful, accurate information, it is of questionable value.

FAQ2 When should I use cytology in practice, and when should I submit specimens to a specialist cytology service?

The following points should be considered:

- Is my time best used for this purpose (cytologic evaluation) or for other techniques? Need to consider economics, customer service, and existing needs within your practice.
- Do I have sufficient training, practice, and interest consistently to obtain specimens of diagnostic quality?
- Do I have sufficient interest and training, or time to devote to training, in order to prepare and stain specimens of diagnostic quality and to have reasonable confidence in my interpretations?
- Do I have a good quality microscope to use? (See also FAQ14)
- What is the availability of a cytologist/cytopathologist? Do I have a good relationship with a cytologist/cytopathologist whom I trust and like?

Reasons to have cytology preparations and stains available, whether or not you use a cytologist/cytopathologist's services, include:

- Confirmation of cellularity of the specimen and likely adequacy of collection, enabling repeated sampling if few or no cells are identified.
- Ability to report preliminary results to owner if immediately prepared.
- Enhance learning of cytologic interpretation by comparison with cytologist/cytopathologist's results.
- Enhance clinical investigative abilities and differential diagnoses by comparison of clinical considerations and cytologic results.

Good reasons for using a cytologist/cytopathologist's services include:
- External confirmation of clinical suspicions and concerns.
- Utilization of expertise and training of a specialist in cytologic evaluation.
- Provision of 'added value' to client service (i.e. consultation with a specialist).
- Possible availability of special stains, concentrating techniques, immunologic staining, etc., which may aid in diagnosis and/or prognosis.

FAQ3 What is considered essential for a good cytology preparation?

Essentials for good cytology preparations include:

Appropriate collection materials and/or devices:
- Usually a 21–25 gauge needle and 5–10 ml syringe are appropriate for fine needle aspiration of cutaneous masses or lesions or body fluids.
- A tuberculin or 25 gauge needle without a syringe is suitable for needle sampling without aspiration. Particularly beneficial for superficial lesions or samples that may exhibit increased cellular fragility, such as enlarged lymph nodes.
- Special holders or devices may be of benefit in improving dexterity and cellularity of specimens.
- Scalpel blades of varying sizes and types may be needed for scrapings.
- Swabs should be dampened with saline or transport medium prior to cell collection in order to prevent dehydration and distortion of cells.
- Some specimens (e.g. bone marrow and CSF) require special needles with a stylet.

Clean, high-quality slides:
- Oil residue can be removed by immersion in alcohol and wiping with lint-free tissue prior to preparing smears. Slides should be dry prior to putting material onto the slide.
- Frosted end slides preferred for ease of labeling and identification.
- If volume permits, multiple slides are preferred in order to increase probability of representative specimen.
- Keep slides covered to prevent accumulation of dust and other air-borne material.

Rapid air drying (hair dryer is useful):
- Prevents 'balling up' (poor spreading of the cell with dark staining) of cells that hinders identification and evaluation of nuclear and cytoplasmic features.
- Rapid air drying promotes optimal cell spreading, prevention of artifacts, and adherence to the slide.

Problem-solving techniques:
- If the specimen is highly viscous and difficult to spread, consider expulsion of material into a small drop of serum or plasma prior to smearing. Will require attention to rapid air drying since serum or plasma will retard air drying.

- Anticoagulant (usually EDTA or sodium citrate) should be available in case bloody specimens or specimens that clot are obtained on initial attempt.

Suitable tubes or holders for transport and submission of specimens:
- Fixative (40% ethanol or 10% buffered formalin) may be suitable for some types of specimens and if appropriate staining techniques (e.g. Papanicolaou, H&E, New Methylene Blue) are used.
- Slide holders should be used to protect smears from dust and dirt and to prevent breakage.
- Protect air-dried smears from formalin fumes that may interfere with staining by Romanowsky methods.

FAQ4 How should I collect cytology specimens?

Fine needle aspirate

Advantages:
- Suitable for sampling many types of cutaneous masses or lesions.
- Usually does not require sedation or anesthesia. Minimal sedation or anesthesia may be required in special cases.

Disadvantages:
- Certain types of lesions may exfoliate poorly on aspiration, especially fibrotic lesions or some tumors of mesenchymal origin.
- Overenthusiastic aspiration may result in blood contamination or hemodilution.

Technique:
- 21–25 gauge needle and 5–10 ml syringe usually adequate.
- Redirect multiple times within the mass in order to increase probability of representative specimen.
- Discontinue suction prior to withdrawal.
- Detach syringe and draw in several milliliters of air.
- Reattach syringe to needle and gently expel material onto labeled glass slides.
- Smear and air dry rapidly (hair dryer).

Ultra-fine needle sampling without aspiration

Advantages:
- Preserves morphology of fragile cells.
- Minimizes or eliminates blood contamination and hemodilution.
- Particularly good for superficial masses and those that may contain fragile cells such as lymph nodes.

Disadvantages:
- Not suitable for deep lesions.
- Not suitable for lesions that exfoliate poorly without aspiration.

Technique:
- Tuberculin or 25 gauge needle usually used.
- 'Stick' mass several times and in multiple areas to obtain a 'core' of representative cells within the needle.
- May see material within hub of needle.
- Withdraw needle.
- Attach syringe containing several milliliters of air.
- Gently expel material onto labeled glass slides.
- Smear and air dry rapidly (hair dryer).

Scraping

Advantages:
- Appropriate for identification of mites and ringworm.
- Some types of lesions that may exfoliate poorly may be adequately sampled by scraping.
- Suitable for ulcerated lesions.

Disadvantages:
- Requires relatively 'deep' scraping to increase probability of representative cells and not just exudate associated with an ulcer.
- May be prone to 'thick' areas containing poorly separated cells that are difficult to interpret.

Technique:
- Use sterile scalpel blade.
- Smear material onto labeled glass slide(s).
- Can make 'squash' preparation to facilitate separation of cells.
- Thin spreads may be facilitated by addition of a small amount of serum or plasma.
- Air dry rapidly (hair dryer).

Imprint

Advantages:
- Usually low probability of information unless done from cut surface of a biopsy.
- Tend to represent surface inflammation, hemorrhage, and/or contamination without inclusion of material representative of deeper cells and processes.
- May be useful for demonstration of superficial yeast (*Malassezia*) or other organisms (usually bacteria).

Disadvantage:
- Not appropriate for most ulcerated or nonulcerated masses.

Technique:
- Gentle wiping with gauze may be of benefit in removing superficial crust or debris that would prevent exfoliation of underlying cells.
- Gently touch surface of labeled slide to area of interest.

- If abundant material is obtained, a 'squash' preparation is suitable. If only a small amount of material, no additional smearing is needed.
- Air dry rapidly (hair dryer).
- Examination of crusts and superficial material may be of benefit in identifying some types of processes.

Swab

Advantages:
- Appropriate for evaluation of exudates or exploration of sinus tracts or draining lesions.
- May be helpful in obtaining material from vesicles or pustules.

Disadvantage:
- Not appropriate for most ulcerated or nonulcerated masses.

Technique:
- Dampen swab with sterile saline or transport medium prior to collection in order to prevent cell dehydration, lysis, and distortion.
- Gently roll swab along slide to dislodge cells.
- Air dry rapidly (hair dryer).

'Scratch and sniff' preparations from biopsies

Advantages:
- May provide more representative material than imprints.
- Useful for rapid evaluation and for 'learning' cytology from corresponding histologic description and diagnosis.

Disadvantages:
- Best preparations obtained from unfixed tissue (suitable for Romanowsky stains) or tissue that has not been in formalin for >12 hours (suitable for Papanicolaou, Trichrome, and H&E stains or wet mounts).
- Cells obtained from tissue in fixative for longer periods of time may not adhere to glass slide, may 'ball up', or may not stain optimally, depending on stain type used.

Technique:
- Identify likely representative area of biopsy.
- Sample from several areas to increase probability of representative cells.
- Use one corner of a clean slide to gently 'scratch' the surface of the biopsy.
- Transfer material from corner of the slide to another slide surface.
- 'Squash' preparations are usually best.
- If rubbery consistency or poor spreading, addition of a small amount of serum may facilitate making thin spreads.
- Air dry rapidly (hair dryer) if Romanowsky stains are to be used. If non-Romanowsky stains (Trichrome, Papanicolaou, H&E) are to be used, cytofixative spray without air drying is recommended.
- Treat appropriately if other stains are to be used.

Washing or lavage

Advantages:
- May provide collection from a wide area or from tubular organs such as lung or reproductive tract.
- May be more sensitive than swab or focal collections.

Disadvantage:
- Requires careful definition of 'adequacy' or 'representativeness' of specimens.

Technique:
- Varies with site and/or species.
- See literature and textbooks for descriptions of washing and lavage collection.

Aspiration of body fluids

Advantages:
- Suitable for abdominal fluid, pleural fluid, pericardial fluid, synovial fluid, and CSF.
- May provide therapeutic advantage by removal of excess fluid with effusions.
- May provide information about processes shedding diagnostic cells or elements into body fluids.

Disadvantage:
- May not reflect underlying pathologic processes, resulting in excess fluid accumulation.

Technique:
- Varies with site and/or species.
- See literature and textbooks for descriptions of collection technique.

FAQ5 How should I prepare my cytology specimens?

A variety of methods can be used depending on the type of specimen and the cellularity. A summary of the type of presentation and techniques and comments regarding the presentations is shown below.

   Direct smears. Suitable for most aspirates of cutaneous masses. Concentration of cells may be needed for specimens of low cellularity.

Blood smear technique

Technique:
- Same as that used for blood smear preparation.
- Drop of specimen is placed at one end of slide.
- Pull end of second slide into the drop at an approximately 45° angle.
- Push portion of drop toward the end of the slide to create a smear that extends approximately three-quarters of the length of the slide and has a feather edge.

Comments:
- Blood smear technique is appropriate for bloody specimens, specimens that are predominantly 'liquid', or specimens that can be expelled into a small drop of serum.
- Larger cells or cell clumps are likely to be concentrated at edges of smear and along feather edge.
- Use of a 'spreader slide' with rounded or angled corners is helpful in producing a smear that is slightly narrower than the width of the slide.
- Spreader slide should be cleaned carefully after use to remove any residual cells and prevent accumulation of dried material that may cause uneven spreading of cell film.

'Pull apart' smears or 'squash' preparations

Technique:
- This technique is the one preferred by the authors for most direct smears.
- Material is gently expelled onto a slide.
- A second slide is placed on top of the first slide and its weight is allowed to spread or 'squash' the material. Sometimes, gentle pressure is needed to promote spreading on the material between the slides.
- The slides are slid apart or 'pulled apart', resulting in cells being smeared on both slides.
- Smears should not travel over the edge of the slide and should not be too close to the edge of the slide.

Comments:
- Care should be taken to prevent excessive pressure on the top slide; this may result in rupture or smudging of cells.
- Some types of rubbery specimens or specimens that are of thick consistency may benefit from expulsion into a small drop of serum or plasma to aid the spreading.
- Gentle circular motions of the top slide may help 'break up' or spread thick accumulations of material or cells.
- Excessive dilution by serum, fluid, or blood may result in migration of cells to the edges of the slide. Carefully observe spreading of the droplet prior to pulling slide apart to prevent loss of cells.

'Line' smears

Technique:
- These smears are made in the same way as the blood smear technique, but instead of completing the smear to form a feather edge, the spreader slide is lifted vertically prior to formation of a feather edge. This results in concentration of cells along a 'line' where the smear is interrupted.

Comment:
- Suitable for the same types of specimens as for blood smear technique.

'Star' spreads

Technique:
- This is the authors' 'least favorite' method of presentation, but it can produce nice presentations when done expertly.
- Material is expelled onto a slide as a droplet.
- A needle or syringe cap is drawn through the droplet in a configuration like that of drawing a five- or six-pointed star.
- This produces a central thick area with thinner 'arms' of the star radiating from it.

Comments:
- Suitable for fluid specimens or for specimens for which the blood smear technique cannot be used.
- Often results in the majority of cells remaining in the central 'thick' area; may be impossible or difficult to evaluate.
- Rapid air drying is more difficult to achieve due to the uneven thickness of the preparation.

Indirect smears. These types of preparations require concentration of cells. Suitable for specimens of low cellularity, specimens in which there is blood or other fluid components, or specimens that are added to a small volume of sterile bacterial transport medium or saline containing 10% serum.

Centrifugation

Technique:
- Gentle centrifugation of specimens that are fluid, contain blood, or have been added to a small quantity of sterile bacterial transport medium or saline containing 10% serum is used to concentrate cells in a pellet at the bottom of the tube.
- Centrifugation equipment and speeds as used for urinalysis and/or separation of serum are appropriate for cell concentration.
- Supernatant is decanted or aspirated.
- Cells are resuspended in a small amount of the fluid remaining in the tube or are aspirated directly from the pellet using a small disposable pipette.
- The cell suspension droplet is transferred to a slide.
- A smear is made by spreading the material with the pipette or by a 'pull apart' or 'squash' technique, depending on the amount of material that is present.

Comments:
- Use of conical tubes facilitates pelleting of sample and easy retention of cells following supernatant decanting. Cells can be resuspended in the small amount of fluid remaining after decanting.

- Concentration by centrifugation is helpful for specimens of low cellularity that may not be easily evaluated in a direct smear preparation.
- If no 'pellet' of cells is visible following centrifugation, special concentration techniques should be considered.

Special concentration techniques
- Special concentration techniques are not likely to be available in most practices. They are more commonly available in large referral practices or in laboratories that specialize in cytologic preparations.
- Special concentration techniques that may be encountered include cytocentrifugation, membrane filtration techniques, thin-prep techniques, and/or sedimentation chambers.

FAQ6 What stains should I use for cytology specimens?

The stains commonly used for cytology specimens are:

Romanowsky stains:
- Diff-Quik®. **NB:** Stains some mast cell granules in mast cell tumors very poorly.
- Wright–Giemsa.
- Other Quik stains.

Wet mounts:
- New Methylene Blue

Stains requiring wet fixation:
- Papanicolaou or Trichrome (some rehydration protocols described for use with air-dried smears).
- Hematoxylin and Eosin.

Commonly used 'special stains':
- Gram stain for gram-negative and gram-positive bacteria.
- Ziehl–Neelsen (acid-fast) stain for acid-fast bacteria.
- Prussian Blue stain for iron.

Romanowsky stains are those most commonly used in practice. There are a number of rapid stains, of which Diff-Quik® is the most well known. Consistency in application and standardization of staining times are important for achieving good quality, consistent results. Try several different timings in order to pick the one with the best nuclear and cytoplasmic contrast. Be prepared to stain lymph node aspirates and bone marrow aspirates for approximately twice the time used for fluids or routine aspirates. Try the routine timing and see if the stain is adequate. If not, the smears can be run through the stain again in an attempt to achieve better staining.

Stain maintenance is an important part of quality control and ensuring that consistent results are obtained.

Stain maintenance and quality control:
- Protect from sunlight.
- Keep covered when not in use.
- Filter periodically (coffee filters are an inexpensive source and acceptable for most stains).
- Clean jars frequently to prevent accumulation of precipitate, growth of organisms, and 'floaters' (cells or organisms that may be within stain and 'float' onto and adhere to a smear; not a true reflection of the lesion, but may contribute to a misdiagnosis).
- Replace stains as indicated by storage, volume of smears, and other conditions.
- Know the stain and its capabilities with regard to colors, transparency, and differentiation.
- Standardize staining times and procedures.
- Know possible artifacts produced by aging of the stain.
- Know possible artifacts produced by nonadherence to standard operating procedures.
- Can use buccal smears (cells scraped from the inside of your cheek) as control smears periodically to evaluate staining adequacy, quality, and technique.
- Know the 'contaminants' associated with your practice: leave slide on bench top during the day and/or overnight in order to accumulate air-borne contaminants.

FAQ7 What are the advantages and disadvantages of using a stain for fixed specimens (e.g. Papanicolaou, Sano's modification of Pollack's Trichrome, or Hematoxylin and Eosin)?

These stains are traditionally used on fixed specimens. Fixation is helpful in preventing cellular degeneration, metabolism, and maturation and in preventing bacterial overgrowth *in vitro*. The nuclear detail provided by these stains is superior because it uses hematoxylin (the same stain as used on tissue sections). The staining characteristics and hues differ from traditional Romanowsky stains and may require experience to identify subtle changes. Bacteria may be more difficult to identify than in Romanowsky-stained smears, particularly when present in small numbers. There are some rapid versions of these stains available, but Romanowsky stains are more commonly used in private practice. These stains may be available in some commercial laboratories. Check with your preferred reference laboratory for the possible availability of these stains and techniques.

FAQ8 What should I expect or include in a cytology report?

The format for a cytology report can vary between laboratories and according to individual preferences. The commonly encountered sections of a cytology report are listed below:

Summary of clinical information:
• May or may not be included.
• In the authors' opinion it is useful to summarize pertinent clinical information about the case.
• Provides a record of the information available at the time of the original interpretation, which may be useful if a second opinion is obtained or smears are reviewed at a later time.

Description:
• May or may not include macroscopic features (color, transparency, character, and macroscopic content). A macroscopic description is useful for determining the classification of the specimen and evaluating the quality of the smears and likelihood of representativeness of the specimen.
• Should include microscopic features.
• Even if pathologists disagree in the interpretation of findings, the description should be similar!

Interpretation:
• Interpretation of findings – should be as specific as the confidence of the reporting cytologist/cytopathologist allows.

Comments:
• Should address the degree of confidence associated with the cytologic interpretation.
• May include differential diagnoses (if appropriate).
• Etiology (if identifiable).
• Prognosis.
• Client education (e.g. expected biological behavior, additional testing or monitoring recommendations, other).
• Address questions or aspects of clinical significance.
• Include other tests or procedures that may be helpful in obtaining a more definitive diagnosis, further definition of the condition, and/or planning for treatment (e.g. T and B cell immunophenotyping, serology, bone marrow aspiration, clinical chemistry, etc.).
• Monitoring that may be appropriate (e.g. regional lymph nodes, local recurrence, multiple tumors).
• Other recommendations (treatment considerations [if knowledgeable], etc.).

FAQ9 What types of cytology specimens should be referred to an experienced cytologist?

The following should be considered for referral to an experienced cytologist:
- All specimens (?).
- Specimens about which you have a question.
- Inflammatory lesions that have not responded to treatment.
- For a second opinion in cases that have a poor prognosis or unusual or unexpected findings.

FAQ10 If a cytology specimen does not provide good information or is not representative, is it worth repeating?

In many instances an initial unsatisfactory specimen or nonspecific findings may be due to the nature of the lesion. Some types of lesion exfoliate poorly on aspiration or may result in nonspecific features. However, in general, evaluation of additional collections may be helpful in:
- Increasing the probability of detection and/or diagnosis of abnormality.
- Increasing the confidence in interpretation if persistent and/or progressive features are identified.
- Increasing the confidence in negative findings, if repeatable.

FAQ11 How do I know if I have a suitable or satisfactory specimen for interpretation, and that it is representative of the lesion?

This is a question that plagues all cytologists. The suitability of a specimen for interpretation will depend on the type of lesion aspirated. General guidelines for various types of cytologic specimen are shown below:

Fine needle aspirates of skin masses or internal masses:
- Usually considered satisfactory/suitable for interpretation if nucleated cells are present. A specimen that does not contain nucleated cells is unsatisfactory or inconclusive. Excessive hemodilution may obscure cells or details or may result in a nonrepresentative specimen.
- Some types of lesion are characterized by low cellularity (e.g. lipomas); other types of lesion (often of mesenchymal origin) may exfoliate poorly on aspiration.

Lymph node aspirate:
- Expected to contain cells of lymphoid origin.
- Sometimes, a lymph node will be totally effaced by inflammation or malignancy. In cases in which lymphoid cells are not present, lymph node involvement cannot be confirmed or ruled out.

Tracheal or bronchial washing:
- Must have cells from several levels of the respiratory tract (columnar and/or cuboidal epithelial cells; macrophages) to have confidence in representation of all levels of the lung.
- Sometimes, a limited interpretation is possible if an abnormality is recognized despite the absence of cells from several levels of the lung.

Bronchoalveolar lavage:
- Macrophages need to be present in order to be considered representative of small airways and alveoli.
- Other cell types may be present.

Urine:
- The absence of cells may be within normal limits.
- 'No abnormality detected' is the most common interpretation when no cells or infectious agents are present.

Cerebrospinal fluid:
- The absence of cells may be within normal limits.
- 'No abnormality detected' is the most common interpretation when no cells or infectious agents are present.

Synovial fluid:
- Some cells are expected. Normally expect a few small lymphocytes, macrophages, and synoviocytes.
- Sometimes other cell types may predominate, depending on the condition that is present.

Pleural and abdominal fluid:
- Some cells expected. Normally expect a mixture of neutrophils and macrophages, with or without a few lymphocytes.
- Sometimes other cell types may predominate, depending on the condition that is present.

Bone marrow aspirate:
- Marrow particles and hematopoietic precursors are needed for optimal interpretation.
- Limited interpretation may be possible if some hematopoietic cells are present, even without marrow particles.

Uterine washing:
- Normally expect epithelial cells. Rare neutrophils and macrophages may be within normal limits. Epithelial morphology differs, depending on the stage of reproductive activity.
- Sometimes other cell types are present, depending on the condition that is present.

- Optimal interpretation also requires correlation with recurrent/current hematologic findings and other evaluations.

Vaginal smears:
- Epithelial cells expected. Bacteria (normal flora) may or may not be present. Remember that aged spayed bitches may have atrophic cuboidal vaginal epithelium and that excessive inflammation or irritation may alter the epithelial morphology and epithelial cell types represented.
- Sometimes other cell types are present, depending on the condition that is present.

Representativeness of a specimen may be difficult to determine. If expected cell types are present in various types of specimen (see above), then there is a high probability that the specimen is representative of the organ or system from which it was obtained. Other factors that need to be taken into account in evaluating whether or not a specimen is likely to be representative of the site of collection include:
- Degree of cellularity.
- Numbers, types, and proportions of cells.
- A bloody specimen may complicate the interpretation of many types of specimen.
- Correlation with the clinical appearance and clinical suspicions about the type of lesion.
- Correlation with the location of the lesion and its suspected significance (e.g. tumor metastatic to lymph node).
- Quality of the specimen (cell preservation and staining).

FAQ12 What if the cytologic evaluation does not fit with the clinical findings or histological interpretation?

In most cases the cytologic findings will correlate well with the clinical findings and histologic evaluation. It is imperative that the cytologic appearance must be correlated with the clinical picture. If it does NOT fit:
- Use good judgement.
- Contact the cytologist for review or send the specimen to an experienced cytologist for a second opinion.
- Consider additional specimens.

Remember, cytologic/histologic correlation is expected with cancer. For some organs/systems (nasal, uterine, respiratory, urinary) the cytologic findings in a lumen may differ from those deeper in the tissue. The degree of correlation may vary with noncancerous conditions. Cytology may vary from histology in representation of cell types and degree of abnormality. The sensitivity, specificity, predictive value of cytology, and histology may vary with site, type of collection, and type of process.

FAQ13 How should I go about evaluating a cytology smear?

The cytologic evaluation should be done in a systematic manner, conducted in the same way each time a slide or set of slides is examined. Initially, the smear should be examined at a low magnification, with special attention at the feather edge (if present), along the edges of the smear, and within the smear to detect unusual features, cells, or groups of cells that may need subsequent examination at a higher magnification.

The low magnification examination will provide information about the overall cellularity and content of the smear and may be helpful in assessing adequacy and representativeness of the specimen, the presentation, and staining. Intermediate magnification is used for the major part of the evaluation to help identify various cell types, their proportions, and their features. High magnification is used to determine fine detail. Additional screening of the smear at low or intermediate magnification, using overlapping fields to cover the entire slide rapidly, may be needed in some cases.

When a cytologic specimen is evaluated, the thought processes of expert evaluators may evolve along different lines, depending on their experience, their training, and their mental organization. However, the following thought processes are identified by most expert evaluators:

- Is the specimen adequate for evaluation? Are the presentation and staining quality adequate?
- Is the specimen likely to be representative of the process or condition in question based on the information about lesion appearance, lesion location, method of collection, and any problems described with that collection (i.e. likely blood contamination)?
- Is the cellularity sufficient for this type of specimen and method of collection?
- Is there any noncellular or background material that may be of significance (i.e. matrix material produced by some mesenchymal tumors, secretory material, necrotic debris that may indicate 'tumor diathesis', lymphoglandular bodies supporting lymphoid tissue origin, cytoplasmic material that may be secretion or phagocytosed material, etc)?
- What numbers, types, and proportions of cells are present?
- Is there a special population of cells that differs from that expected or which should not be present?
- What type of process does this likely represent (i.e. inflammatory, noninflammatory, proliferative, non-neoplastic, neoplastic, benign, or malignant)?
- Can the process be further characterized or subcategorized in a way that will provide useful information (i.e. what type of inflammation; if neoplastic, with what type of tumor or group of tumors is this compatible)?
- Is an etiology apparent (infectious agent, foreign material)?
- If neoplastic, do the cells have features of being benign or malignant?
- If neoplastic, can the cell type of origin be identified specifically or to a particular group or category?

- What degree of confidence is there in the cytologic interpretation of the specimen?
- What is the expected biological behaviour based on these findings?
- Are there additional tests that may be of benefit for confirmation, prognosis, staging, or evaluation of the extent of the disease, or increasing confidence in the interpretation?
- Are there treatments or other recommendations that the cytologist is knowledgeable enough to make about this condition?
- Is there a need for a second opinion or additional research into this case (comparison with cases of known diagnoses, literature search, reference text, etc)?

FAQ14 What kind of microscope is best for cytology evaluations?

In general, a binocular microscope is best. The lenses should include low, medium and high magnifications, usually ×4, ×10, ×20, and ×40, or ×50 oil and ×100 oil. An adjustable light source and condenser should be present in order to provide the appropriate lighting and contrast that are needed at various magnifications and for a variety of specimens.

FAQ15 What is the best way of preserving slides for an archive?

Slides should be stored in a clean, dry environment and protected from light. In order to prevent damage to the surface of the smear, it should be mounted with a coverslip using a mounting medium such as Permount or Eukitt. These are usually xylene-soluble, and xylene can be used to clean oil from the surface of the smear if it has been examined prior to coverslipping. The coverslip should be mounted without air bubbles and allowed to dry flat before storing. The stored slides should be labeled with an indelible marker so that they can be identified for future reference. Slides with a frosted end are particularly useful, since they can be written on in pencil and the pencil will not rub off with storage. A file containing reports or other information corresponding to the smears is useful. Any follow-up information (clinical or histologic) can be included in this file.

FAQ16 How often are infectious agents seen in cytologic specimens?

The frequency with which infectious agents are seen in cytologic specimens will depend on the types of specimens obtained and the conditions most frequently seen in the practice. The absence of infectious agents cytologically does not rule out the possibility of infection. A common cytology teaching adage is: 'the absence of evidence is not evidence of absence'. However, when infections are present, the likelihood of detecting infectious agents is increased when:

- A representative specimen is obtained.
- The specimen is well stained.
- The specimen is examined by a person experienced in the recognition of a variety of infectious agents.

The possibility of false-positive identification of infectious agents also exists. Sometimes, granular precipitate or debris resembles bacteria. If an unfixed specimen is received by post, there may be overgrowth of bacteria from contamination or overgrowth of a pathogen. If fluid specimens are obtained, making a cytologic preparation from the freshly collected specimen with minimal or no delay prior to processing is likely to provide the best sample. If referral laboratories offer special stains for fixed specimens (e.g. Papanicolaou, Sano's modification of Pollack's Trichrome stain, H&E, or a wet mount preparation using New Methylene Blue), then addition of fixative may help prevent or limit bacterial overgrowth during transport to the laboratory. This is particularly important for specimens that may require overnight transport by post or courier. The availability of such stains for fixed specimens will vary with the laboratory. Fixation will also help preserve cellular morphology and prevent the ongoing degeneration, metabolism, or maturation that may occur in unfixed specimens during transport to the laboratory. Check with your referral laboratory for their preferred methods.

The other measures that may be helpful in preventing contamination with infectious agents that would result in false-positive results are:

- Handle specimens only in a clean environment.
- Wash all glassware, pipettes, and other instruments frequently. Disposable plastic pipettes should be used to prevent the contamination that may occur when pipettes are reused.
- Place fluid specimens only in clean tubes.
- Do not leave slides in an unprotected environment that may result in environmental contamination of the slide surface.
- Filter stains frequently and make sure that glassware containing stains is clean and free from precipitate and 'floating material'.
- If it known that a specimen probably contains infectious agents or numerous bacteria or yeast, or if other infectious agents are observed on microscopic examination, filter the stains prior to running other slides through the stain.

A standard coffee filter can be used to filter most cytologic stains. These filters can be reused until such time as they accumulate sufficient material to block the pores and prevent the liquid from coming through the filter. Remember to filter stain only into a clean dry jar.

If infectious agents are suspected in some types of preparations (e.g. wet-mounts or unstained urine sediment), then evaluation of a stained sediment smear may be helpful to confirm this suspicion. The presence of intracellular bacteria provides good support for the presence of sepsis. Extracellular bacteria may also indicate infection, but contaminants or overgrowth should also be considered when extracellular organisms are present.

FAQ17 What if my smears stain too darkly (so darkly that I cannot identify the cells)?

Smears stained too darkly may be due to:
- Excessively thick smears that are not rapidly air dried. This may cause cells to round up (not spread out well) and stain very darkly. Hint: a hand-held hair drier or warming plate may be used on a low setting to help dry smears rapidly.
- Excessive staining times in one or more of the solutions with manual staining.
- Presence of excessive mucus or other secretion that may obscure cells and/or contribute to slow air drying.

FAQ18 What do I do if my smears stain very blue, without much contrast between nucleus and cytoplasm?

Excessive blue staining may be due to:
- Excessive time in the blue stain or too little time in the red/orange stain if using a manual stain. Check that the red/orange stain has not been exhausted when it appears that the staining time is within the expected limits.
- Exposure to formalin fumes. This is why specimens in formalin should be packaged separately from air-dried smears for Romanowsky staining. Air-dried smears for Romanowsky staining should not be handled or prepared in a poorly ventilated area where formalin is also present.
- Incorrect pH of the stains or water.

FAQ19 What should I do if the smear is obscured by clumps of stain precipitate?

- Filter the stains. Be sure to filter into a clean jar.
- Clean out the staining jars (use 3% bleach solution to remove any stubborn precipitate staining with scrubbing).
- Make sure that smears are being rinsed properly. If tap water is used, make sure it is not excessively hard water (may need to use distilled water or a water softener on the water supply).

FAQ20 What should I do if my lymph node and bone marrow aspirates, in particular, stain very pale?

These types of preparation may need adjustments to the staining times. With manual staining, you may need to lengthen the staining times (double or triple). If using an automatic stainer, you may want to run the slides through the stainer twice. This may help improve the quality of the staining, but will not be effective for all slides. Sometimes, a wet preparation (can be done on top of the poorly stained smear) with a drop of New Methylene Blue under a coverslip will be helpful. However, sometimes you just have to do the best you can with the pale staining!

FAQ21 How do I know if my Romanowsky staining is adequate?

The purpose of staining is to provide contrast and differentiation of cells and their structures at the light microscopic level. The Romanowsky stains are a group of stains that contain methylene blue and/or the products of its oxidation and a halogenated fluorescein dye, usually Eosin B or Y. These stains are referred to as 'polychrome stains' because they can result in a range of colors, known as the 'Romanowsky effect'. Staining with Romanowsky stains is influenced by the proportions of the various stains and oxidation production, buffer used, buffer pH, staining time, and removal of excess stain.

To have adequate staining, air-dried smears should contain a monolayer of cells. The cells should be spread out so they are not quite touching and rapidly air dried so that they spread out on the surface of the glass. Use of a control smear (see FAQ26 on control for cytology) may be helpful in ensuring that the quality of staining is adequate.

With a Romanowsky stain, good staining is characterized by the ability to see the nucleus in nucleated cells, which should be purple to blue, with clear definition of its chromatin and nucleoli (if present). The cytoplasmic boundaries of cells should be evident so that you can determine the size and shape of the cell. Cytoplasm may stain a variety of colors, depending on the cell type and its contents. Pink–orange eosinophil granules should be identifiable. Mast cell granules may stain variably (not at all, poorly, or well), depending on the Romanowsky stained used.

FAQ22 What classification should be used for pleural and abdominal fluid specimens, and how is it helpful?

The classical approach to classification of pleural and abdominal fluid specimens is to use NCC and TP to determine if the fluid is likely to be a transudate, a modified transudate, or an exudate. Other classifications may be based on the cytologic findings, including hemorrhagic effusions, neoplastic effusions, nonspecific effusions, pyothorax, pyoabdomen, or septic effusions. All classification schemes have drawbacks, since there are some specimens that do not fit nicely into the various classifications provided. The traditional classification system based on NCC and TP may provide a good starting point for consideration of those conditions that commonly cause these findings. The cytologic appearance may or may not provide a likely cause, but it can help determine the best approach for continued investigation or treatment of the condition.

Transudates are classically associated with hypoproteinemia/hypoalbuminemia. Usually, albumin is <15–18 g/l (1.5–1.8 g/dl) before effusion will form due to decreased osmotic colloidal pressure alone. Transudates may also be seen with early cardiac insufficiency or other noninflammatory causes of effusions.

Exudates are most often seen with inflammatory or infectious conditions, but may also occur with neoplastic or lymphocytic effusions that are the result of lymph stasis. Lymph stasis may be associated with cardiac insufficiency or the presence of an internal mass or chylous effusion that is interfering with venous/lymphatic return.

Modified transudates are effusions with intermediate characteristics that may include a variety of underlying causes. The prognosis for these conditions is often poor, since modified transudates are often associated with malignancy or conditions involving organs or systems that are not easily resolved.

FAQ23 What should I do if all I get is a very bloody specimen (effusion or aspirate)?

Remember that the leukocytes usually will be present in this type of preparation. Sometimes, only erythrocytes will be present as a result of contamination, but often leukocytes are present in the numbers, types, and proportions present in the peripheral blood. Platelets (if present) will also be concentrated. Examine carefully for hemic and nonhemic cell types.

- Make a buffy coat smear to try to concentrate the nucleated cells. The procedure for making a buffy coat smear is as follows:
  - Fill several microhematocrit tubes with a well-mixed specimen and spin as you would to obtain a PCV.
  - With a file, score just BELOW the buffy coat (whitish layer on top of the RBC column).
  - Carefully break the tube and gently tap to expel the buffy coat onto a slide. If the material does not come out of the tube with gentle tapping, an unbent paper clip can be inserted into the tube to push the material out gently and onto a slide.
  - Make a 'squash preparation' or blood smear type preparation.
  - Rapidly air dry.
  - Stain with a Romanowsky stain.

FAQ24 What are the cytologic criteria for malignancy?

The following criteria are commonly associated with malignancy. Each by itself, or in some combination, may occur with stimulation of cells associated with hyperplasia or dysplasia or, in some cases, with inflammation. If the criteria are consistently present and multiple criteria are present, then malignancy is more likely. The criteria include:

- Uneven chromatin distribution.
- Increased chromatin clumping or prominence.
- Nucleoli or macronucleoli (volume of the nucleolus is more than or equal to 50% of the volume of the nucleus) – may be single or multiple.
- Irregularly shaped (not round) nucleoli.
- Increased N:C ratio.
- Mitotic figures, especially if asymmetrical.
- Multinucleation.
- Abnormal variation in cellular size (anisocytosis).
- Abnormal variation in nuclear size (anisokaryosis).
- Inappropriate cell type or appearance for the site of collection (rule out spurious collection from local tissues first).
- Uneven nuclear membrane thickening or clumping of chromatin along the nuclear membrane.
- Nuclear molding.
- Cellular anaplasia (lack of differentiation).
- Cytoplasmic development uncoordinated with or inappropriate for the nuclear features.

FAQ25 How can I increase confidence in interpretation of malignancy and differentiation of malignant from nonmalignant features?

Confidence can be increased with experience and feedback. Features that help increase confidence in the presence of malignancy are:

- Large numbers of atypical cells that exhibit cytologic criteria of malignancy.
- Monomorphic population of cells that is not complicated by a variety of cell types.
- Asymmetric mitotic figures.

It is harder to be confident if malignant cells are few, the overall cellularity is not high, or if features of malignancy are subtle.

Comparison with the results of histology (if available) provides the best feedback. Correlation with clinical progression may be helpful in cases in which tissue confirmation is not available. Comparison with a report written by an experienced cytologist can also provide good feedback and an opportunity to learn.

With the advent of digital microscopic photography, which can be transmitted via e-mail and the internet, it is possible to transmit images so that questions about particular cells or features can be analyzed and information shared amongst cytologists. Although photographic images may not provide the same total picture as examination of the glass slide, they may provide valuable illustrations of significant features and may be very useful as a learning tool.

FAQ26 What can I use for a control in cytology?

A control is a standard material or item used to characterize performance of a method. For cytology, common types of smears used for controls can be a blood smear, a buffy coat smear made from the WBC layer in a microhematocrit tube, or a buccal scraping (scraping from the inside of your cheek that is smeared on a slide).

You can use one or more of the 'control smears' to determine if your cytology stain is working well and providing enough contrast and differentiation. If you examine one or more control smears periodically, this is a good check on the ongoing quality of staining. It helps to examine a control smear frequently enough to be confident in the interpretation of 'good staining'. This might range from once per week to twice a month. A control smear also should be examined anytime that you have changed one or more of the solutions used for staining or if you have a question about whether unusual staining observed with a patient sample is the result of the sample itself or a problem with the stain.

FAQ27 How do I go about evaluating a cytology slide?

A systematic approach to slide examination is considered crucial in the correct interpretation of cytologic samples. With poor examination technique, a lack of recognition of important details and a tendency to examine the slide at high-power field immediately or too quickly are only a couple of the errors that can easily lead to a wrong diagnosis and/or incorrect clinical decisions. Smears should be initially scanned with low-power objective ($\times 4$–$\times 10$) to gain an appreciation of the overall cellularity and the preservation.

Preservation is also essential for a correct cytologic interpretation and usually requires observation at higher magnification ($\times 20$–$\times 40$). The presence of intact cells with clearly recognizable cytoplasmic borders and nuclear details reflect good cellular preservation. When a smear is characterized by high numbers of disrupted cells without clear and distinct cytoplasm (bare nuclei, naked nuclei) cytologic interpretation is not possible.

Without intact, well-preserved cells there is a probability that the cytologic preparation will be nondiagnostic and, therefore, re-collection should be considered.

Assuming the cellularity and the preservation of the sample are adequate, the next step is the evaluation of the main cell type present in the smears.

The prevalence of inflammatory cells (e.g. neutrophils, eosinophils, lymphocytes, monocytes/macrophages) is supportive of an inflammatory process; the presence of a significant number of other cell types (e.g. epithelial, mesenchymal, or round cells) is usually seen in hyperplastic/dysplastic/neoplastic conditions of different origins. Interestingly, coexistence of both inflammatory and neoplastic cells is not uncommon since rapidly growing tumors may easily cause tissue necrosis and, therefore, concurrent inflammation secondary to this. Skin tumors (especially squamous cell carcinoma) may ulcerate, leading to a concurrent inflammation, which sometimes may also be septic.

Additional reading

Cowell RL, Tyler RD (2002) (eds) *Diagnostic Cytology and Hematology of the Horse*, 2nd edn. Mosby, St. Louis.

Fournel-Fleury C, Magnol JP, Guelfi JF (1994) (eds) *Color Atlas of Cancer Cytology of the Dog and Cat*. Pratique Médicale et Chirurgicale de l'Animal de Compagnie, Paris.

Harvey JW (2012) (eds) *Veterinary Hematology: a Diagnostic Guide and Color Atlas*. Saunders, Elsevier, St. Louis.

Raskin RE, Meyer DJ (2016) (eds) *Atlas of Canine and Feline Cytology*, 3rd edn). Saunders, Elsevier, St. Louis.

Thrall MA, Weiser G, Allison L, Campbell TW (2004) (eds) *Veterinary Hematology and Clinical Chemistry*, 2nd edn. Wiley-Blackwell, Ames.

Valenciano AC, Cowell RL (2014) (eds) *Cowell and Tyler's Diagnostic Cytology and Hematology of the Dog and Cat*, 4th edn. Mosby, Elsevier, St. Louis.

Villiers E, Ristic J (2016) (eds) *BSAVA Manual of Canine and Feline Clinical Pathology*, 3rd edn. British Small Animal Veterinary Association, Gloucester.

Weiss DJ, Wardrop KJ (2010) (eds) *Schalm's Veterinary Hematology*, 6th edn. Wiley-Blackwell, Ames.

Withrow SJ, Vail DM, Page R (2013) (eds) *Small Aimal Clinical Oncology*, 5th edn. Saunders, Elsevier, St. Louis.

Index

Note: References are to case numbers, not page numbers.

Also available in the Self-Assessment Color Review series

Brown & Rosenthal: *Small Mammals*
Elsheikha & Patterson: *Veterinary Parasitology*
Forbes & Altman: *Avian Medicine & Surgery 2nd Edition*
Freeman: *Veterinary Cytology*
Frye: *Reptiles and Amphibians 2nd Edition*
Hartmann & Levy: *Feline Infectious Diseases*
Hartmann & Sykes: *Canine Infectious Diseases*
Keeble, Meredith & Richardson: *Rabbit Medicine and Surgery 2nd Edition*
Kirby, Rudloff & Linklater: *Small Animal Emergency and Critical Care Medicine 2nd Edition*
Lewbart: *Ornamental Fishes and Aquatic Invertebrates 2nd Edition*
Lewis & Langley-Hobbs: *Small Animal Orthopedics, Rheumatology & Musculoskeletal Disorders 2nd Edition*
Mair & Divers: *Equine Internal Medicine 2nd Edition*
May & McIlwraith: *Equine Orthopaedics and Rheumatology*
Meredith & Keeble: *Wildlife Medicine and Rehabilitation*
Moriello: *Small Animal Dermatology*
Moriello & Diesel: *Small Animal Dermatology, Advanced Cases*
Obradovich: *Small animal Clinical Oncology*
Pycock: *Equine Reproduction and Stud Medicine*
Samuelson & Brooks: *Small Animal Ophthalmology*
Scott: *Cattle and Sheep Medicine 2nd Edition*
Sparkes & Caney: *Feline Medicine*
Tennant: *Small Animal Abdominal and Metabolic Disorders*
Thieman-Mankin: *Small Animal Soft Tissue Surgery 2nd Edition*
Verstraete & Tsugawa: *Veterinary Dentistry 2nd Edition*
Ware: *Small Animal Cardiopulmonary Medicine*